THE LAST TEN POUNDS

THE LAST TEN POUNDS

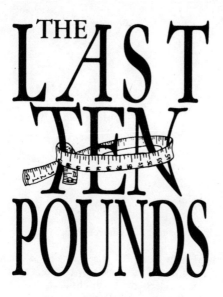

The Diet to Finally Lose Them!

Linda Konner

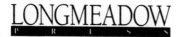

LONGMEADOW
PRESS

Jacket design by Hannah Lerner
Interior design by Hannah Lerner

Library of Congress Catologing-in-Publication Data

Konner, Linda.
    The last 10 pounds : the diet to finally lose them / Linda
Konner.
        p.   cm.
    ISBN 0-681-41193-7
    1. Reducing.   2. Body image.   I. Title.   II. Title: Last ten
pounds.
RM222.2.K577   1991
613.2'5—dc20   91-35134
                                                          CIP

Printed in United States of America
First Edition

0 9 8 7 6 5 4 3 2 1

*For David,
who has cheered me on,
through thin and thick,
for 20 years.*

ACKNOWLEDGMENTS

A special thanks to the following people for their information, time, and support during the writing of this book: Calvin Konner, April Koral, Judy Marshel, Diane Milhan, Tony van der Meer, and, of course, my honey Peter.

AUTHOR'S NOTE

This book is not intended to be a medical manual. If you believe you have a medical problem, see a doctor. Also, remember that nutrition and health needs vary from person to person, depending on age, sex, and overall health. The information provided here is intended to help you make intelligent decisions if you decide to lose weight, but should not be a substitute for any treatment that may have been prescribed for you by your physician. Consult your doctor before embarking on any weight-loss program suggested in this book.

CONTENTS

THE LAST TEN POUNDS

INTRODUCTION

• Are you one of those people who *always* has "just 10 more pounds to go"?

• Are you forever agonizing over whether to eat even that extra one-ounce piece of broiled salmon, for fear you'll blow your diet?

• Are friends and relatives constantly saying, *"You,* on a diet? You look fine to me" (but you don't believe it for a second)?

• Do you sabotage your own weight-loss efforts by living on Lean Cuisine for five days straight, followed by an intimate weekend with Ben & Jerry (not to mention Sara Lee and Oscar Meyer)—then wonder why you can never seem to drop those last stubborn pounds?

• Do you like yourself only when your bathroom scale gives you permission to do so?

• Do you believe that all those wonderful dreams of yours—a better job/a loving mate/a spiffy wardrobe/a romantic vacation—will somehow come true once you're just a *little* thinner?

These examples may seem like a lot of *different* dieting dilemmas, but they're actually all an offshoot of one: The Last 10 Pounds Syndrome.

It's always the same old story: "Ten pounds more and I'll be happy!" (or five or 15—some relatively small number). And that's the feeling whether you're wearing a size 4 or a 12, even if you're in flawless health, even if you exercise like a demon, even if you're the envy of all your chubby friends. Life will never be worth living—not fully, anyway—until your body precisely fits the standards set by some insurance company's height/weight chart, some celebrity's measurements published in *People* magazine, or your own vision of what is suitably slim.

And so your days are an endless quest for the "perfect" diet, the "perfect" health club, the "perfectly" cut suit (to hide those figure flaws), the "perfect" slimming haircut (to narrow a "wide" face). Meanwhile, everything else is put on hold until the magic moment when the needle on the scale points to *your* ideal weight, that glorious three-digit combination almost as thrilling as a winning lottery number, the one you've been dreaming of seeing again since you were a high-school sophomore.

It's all pretty exhausting, isn't it?

Few people understand and appreciate the agony of constantly being on a diet better than I do. As the former editor-in-chief of *Weight Watchers Magazine,* I've had the opportunity to try every diet technique, from fasting to drinking protein shakes, from snacking on low-calorie chocolate mousse to soaking for hours at a time in an isolation tank. Because I came to the job as a lifelong dieter, I made the perfect guinea . . . uh, pig.

I intend in this book to help you sort the useful from the useless in terms of weight-loss information, as I have learned to do over the years. But *The Last Ten Pounds* has, above all, a message to impart: Your "need" to diet may be mostly in your head. What you may label a weight problem might *really* be an indication of low self-esteem, a desire to shift your focus away from a more unpleasant situation (the lack of a fulfilling relationship, for example)—and even plain old boredom. (Counting calories and exercising for hours on end *do* kill time.)

A "weight problem," whether real or imaginary, is something that's usually been years or even decades in the making; quick-fix cures won't shoo the situation—or the extra pounds—away. With this in mind, *The Last Ten Pounds* will help you explore the *true* roots of your dilemma. Furthermore, you'll be provided with a *variety* of options for dealing with your extra 10 pounds, which, in your particular case, may or may not mean putting yourself on a weight-loss diet. Whatever course of action this pro–choice book helps you select, two outcomes are certain: Your chronic dieting will be a thing of the past, and you'll finally be happy with the body you're in.

I

ARE YOU *REALLY* OVERWEIGHT?

The Last 10 Pounds Quiz

Put down that chicken leg, pick up a pencil, and take this quiz. Really *think* about the questions and your responses. Your answers will help you take a clear-eyed look at your eating patterns and problems, and what your next steps need to be.

1. Once I put my mind to it, I tend to take off weight relatively quickly and easily.
   TRUE _____ FALSE _____

2. I feel like I've been on a diet my whole life.
   TRUE _____ FALSE _____

3. Eating is one of my three all-time favorite activities.
   TRUE _____ FALSE _____

4. People are amazed by my ability to tabulate mentally the calorie counts for everything on my plate.
   TRUE _____ FALSE _____

5. Getting on the scale is usually a terrifying experience.
TRUE _____ FALSE _____

6. I am waiting to ask my boss for a raise (or get married, or some other major change) until I look better (i.e., I'm thinner).
TRUE _____ FALSE _____

7. When I finally meet someone with whom I've had only a telephone relationship, I'm thrilled if I'm thinner than that person.
TRUE _____ FALSE _____

8. I'm pleased with the way I look nude.
TRUE _____ FALSE _____

9. My mate is pleased with the way I look nude.
TRUE _____ FALSE _____

10. I weigh myself more than three times a week.
TRUE _____ FALSE _____

11. When people tell me I look thin, I tend not to believe them.
TRUE _____ FALSE _____

12. When people tell me I look thin, I usually attribute it to the outfit I'm wearing or having just gotten over an acute case of stomach flu.
TRUE _____ FALSE _____

13. I have tried more than four different diets in my life.
TRUE _____ FALSE _____

14. If a genie gave me the chance to maintain my current weight forever (never getting fatter *or* thinner), I'd happily take it.
    TRUE _____ FALSE _____

15. I feel 100 percent better about myself when I'm at my "ideal" weight.
    TRUE _____ FALSE _____

16. I can now wear a bathing suit or shorts without too much self-consciousness.
    TRUE _____ FALSE _____

17. I have deliberately canceled vacation plans in the past because I was embarrassed about showing off my body in warm-weather clothes.
    TRUE _____ FALSE _____

18. I am always the biggest eater in any group.
    TRUE _____ FALSE _____

19. I own more than five diet books.
    TRUE _____ FALSE _____

20. I am satisfied with my level of regular exercise.
    TRUE _____ FALSE _____

21. My doctor usually tells me I should drop 10 pounds or so.
    TRUE _____ FALSE _____

22. I tend to lose interest in my overall appearance when I'm even a little heavier than I'd like to be.
    TRUE _____ FALSE _____

23. I have a hard time enjoying my favorite foods because of the guilt.

    TRUE _____   FALSE _____

24. My weight has seldom interfered with my enjoyment of sex.

    TRUE _____   FALSE _____

25. Boy, this quiz has made me hungry! I could go for a slice of double-cheese pizza right now!

    TRUE _____   FALSE _____

ANSWERS

It would've been simple to come up with the kind of complicated scoring system you usually see in these quizzes. But honestly, after all the diets you've been on and all the quizzes you've taken in your life, you *already* know the score. You *also* know that being aware of the numbers isn't enough. (Has knowing that a slab of cherry cheesecake contains 375 calories ever stopped you from eating it at midnight in the glow of the refrigerator light?)

You may be only 10 pounds over your ideal weight, yet it's enough of an issue for you that you've turned to this book for help. Good.

Illusion vs. Reality,
or, the Perfect-Body Myth

Self-image is the way you see yourself and project yourself to others. It's a perception that's generally based on the way you feel about yourself. For a variety of reasons, simple and complex, some dating back to your infancy and others much more recent, you may have a distorted idea about the way you appear, to those around you and in the mirror. If you're trying to shed the last 10 pounds after a fairly major weight loss, you may still unwittingly be clinging to a "fat" image of yourself. Even if you've never had more than about 10 pounds to lose, you may have grown so accustomed to being constantly on a diet and *feeling* fat that you can't see how close to a healthy weight you truly are.

Yet developing a good self-image, along with reasonable diet expectations, is crucial for people who feel they have 10 pounds to lose. With a realistic self-image in place, you may decide that dieting off those 10 pounds is ultimately unnecessary. And if you insist that those pounds must go, an accurate self-image will let you be sensible about your weight-loss goals and the way your body may (or may not) look in the future.

How do you see yourself? Are you currently measuring yourself against a faded snapshot of yourself at age 18? Against the way your teenage daughter or neighbor looks? Against the image of 23-year-old magazine or department store models? Now's the perfect time for a quick reality check. The following simple exercises were created by Judy Marshel, M.B.A., R.D., director of Health Resources, in Great Neck, New York. They will get you in touch with your mental image of yourself and help you determine whether losing those last 10 pounds is right for you:

1. Leaf through some newspapers and magazines, and pick out the person you'd most like to resemble in terms of body size and type. What about that individual appeals to you so much? In evaluating the age, height, body type, and other physical details of the person you chose, ask yourself: Given who I am—in terms

of my age, height, body type, etc.—is it realistic for me to diet down to that size?

2. Think about your own body in detail—the good, the bad, and everything in between. Ask yourself: How do I look right now? Am I really 10 pounds overweight, or do I just *think* I am? Is it possible that my good areas outweigh the bad?

3. Get a full-size sheet of blank paper and draw an outline of the way you think your body looks. Then scrutinize your nude body in front of a full-length mirror. How accurate is your drawing? Did you depict yourself as much bigger (or smaller) than you really are?

4. Add to your body outline the various parts of your body and try to figure out what they say about your personality. Have you drawn a big heart? Large teeth? A tiny mouth? What are the connections between the image you have of your body and that of your personality?

5. A variation on Exercise 3: Draw your body as you would *like* it to look someday. Then, taking a good look at your nude body, decide how realistic your goal is. Hold on to the drawing and, if you decide to diet, continue to refine it periodically as you lose weight.

6. If you feel comfortable, show your drawings to a good friend. Discuss her reactions. Does she believe they accurately reflect your body? What parts of your body does she think you're exaggerating?

7. Identify the clothing styles and particular garments you favor. Do they make you feel self-confident or self-conscious

about your body? How and why do you think that is? What image
do you hope to project with your clothes?

8. Write an imaginary Personals ad for yourself, focusing first
on your physical characteristics. How would you describe your
height? Weight? Overall body type—voluptuous, slim, Rube-
nesque, statuesque, cuddly? Now write a statement that reflects
your *inner* self. (You're much more than just the way you look.)
Is this a person *you'd* like to meet and get to know?

9. Try positive affirmations (written or verbal statements in the
present tense) and creative visualization (using your imagination
to create what you want). These techniques will help you "see"
yourself as you wish to be, today and in days to come. Constantly
repeat such affirmations as:

- "My body is trim and healthy."
- "My body is attractive to others."
- "I'm taking positive steps to look the way I want to."
- "My body is always improving and looking better."

In addition, conjure up mental pictures of yourself looking slim,
happy, and satisfied. Whether or not you decide to lose the last 10
pounds, these exercises will help you feel better about your body
instantly.

What Do You Like About Your Body?
(There's Got to Be Something)

Complain, complain. Instead of focusing on the 10 pounds you
hate, why not shift your attention to the parts of you that you
love?

Everybody has something she likes about her own body. Which parts of you are pretty nice, or even terrific? Check them off below. (Note: Only take this test while you're in a good mood and/or in a rational frame of mind.)

	GREAT	GOOD	COULD BE GOOD WITH SOME WORK	EH . . ?
Hair				
Eyes				
Nose				
Mouth/smile				
Teeth				
Skin				
Neck				
Arms				
Hands/nails				
Shoulders				
Breasts/chest				
Waist/stomach				
Hips				
Derriere				
Genitals				
Legs				
Feet				

Sure, there are parts you wish you could exchange for one or two of Kim Basinger's or Patrick Swayze's. But don't forget there's still plenty about the body you have that's great to look at and fondle. Just ask the people who love you.

Height/Weight Charts:
Should You Believe Them?

Are you guilty of living your dieting life according to the numbers on those dreary height/weight charts, panicking the minute you happen to gain a pound or two beyond the highest "acceptable" weight for your height, frame, and age? If so, there are a few things you should know about these numbers.

First, they were compiled to serve as human *longevity* statistics, not necessarily "ideal" goal weights for healthy, living people. They were put together by number-crunchers trying to come up with appropriate life-insurance rates. That's not to say they can't be used as a guideline by you, someone concerned with their last 10 pounds. But what you consider 10 pounds of overweight may, as these charts demonstrate, actually be "acceptable," given the wide range within each category.

Second, even these "standard" weights and measures can change—*and have*. For example, if you're still going by the 1959 Metropolitan Life Insurance table, the granddaddy of all the height/weight charts (see page 15), you'll be glad to learn that in 1983 it was revised just the way you like it: *upward* (see pages 16 and 17). That means you can now be several pounds heavier than before and be considered an "acceptable," healthy weight.

According to a Met Life spokeswoman, the new tables were based on studies conducted between 1959 and 1981 by the Society of Actuaries, again based on longevity statistics, not necessarily quality of life. However, as the spokeswoman was quick to point out, "Because there is a fear of overweight people getting life insurance, the numbers were carefully reviewed and the extra pounds added to the charts were not considered a health risk. And . . . the higher weights make people feel a little better about their own." So, for instance, if in 1959 you were a 5'5" medium-framed woman, your "acceptable" weight range was 116–130; today that range is 127–141.

The people at the U. S. Department of Agriculture and U.S. Department of Health and Human Resources are kinder still. *Their* most recent height/weight table allows for even higher weights, particularly if you're 35 or older (see page 18). As the explanation accompanying their chart says, "Recent research suggests that people can be a little heavier as they grow older without added risk to health."

"Health, shmealth!," you might be saying, followed by, "Just *look* at those charts! If I weighed as much as they say I can, I'd be a blimp!" Okay. We *know* people lose and gain weight for reasons that aren't strictly health-related; rightly or wrongly, appearance has much more to do with people's dieting decisions. But if you still think you'd be overweight at the *lowest* end of the range on the height/weight chart, now's a good time to start asking yourself if your weight-loss goals are truly realistic.

Remember, too, that height/weight charts are but one weight-measuring tool. There's also the faithful scale (more on that later), fat-measuring devices, your own medical condition, and—not to be lightly dismissed—the way you feel and look.

So use the height/weight tables you see here as a guideline, or follow whichever others you prefer—or none at all. The choice is yours.

DESIRABLE WEIGHTS FOR MEN AND WOMEN
AGE 25 AND OVER*
(in pounds according to height and frame, in
indoor clothing)

Height		Small Frame	Medium Frame	Large Frame
		Men		
Feet	Inches			
5	2	112–120	118–129	126–141
5	3	115–123	121–133	129–144
5	4	118–126	124–136	132–148
5	5	121–129	127–139	135–152
5	6	124–133	130–143	138–156
5	7	128–137	134–147	142–161
5	8	132–141	138–152	147–166
5	9	136–145	142–156	151–170
5	10	140–150	146–160	155–174
5	11	144–154	150–165	159–179
6	0	148–158	154–170	164–184
6	1	152–162	158–175	168–189
6	2	156–167	162–180	173–194
6	3	160–171	167–185	178–199
6	4	164–175	172–190	182–204
		Women		
4	10	98– 98	96–107	104–119
4	11	94–101	98–110	106–122
5	0	96–104	101–113	109–125
5	1	99–107	104–116	112–128
5	2	102–110	107–119	115–131
5	3	105–113	110–122	118–134
5	4	108–116	113–126	121–138
5	5	111–119	116–130	125–142
5	6	114–123	120–135	129–146
5	7	118–127	124–139	133–150
5	8	122–131	128–143	137–154
5	9	126–135	132–147	141–158
5	10	130–140	136–151	145–163
5	11	134–144	140–155	149–168
6	0	138–148	144–159	153–173

*Adapted from Metropolitan Life Insurance Company., New York. New weight standards for men and women. *Statistical Bulletin 40:3*, November-December, 1959.

1983 Metropolitan Height & Weight Tables

Weights at ages 25-59 based on lowest mortality. Weight in pounds according to frame (in indoor clothing weighing 5 lbs. for men and 3 lbs. for women; shoes with 1" heels).

Metropolitan Life ®
AND AFFILIATED COMPANIES

Metropolitan Life Insurance Company
Health and Safety Education Division

1983 METROPOLITAN HEIGHT AND WEIGHT TABLES*

Men

Height Feet	Inches	Small Frame	Medium Frame	Large Frame
5	2	128–134	131–141	138–150
5	3	130–136	133–143	140–153
5	4	132–138	135–145	142–156
5	5	134–140	137–148	144–160
5	6	136–142	139–151	146–164
5	7	138–145	142–154	149–168
5	8	140–148	145–157	152–172
5	9	142–151	148–160	155–176
5	10	144–154	151–163	158–180
5	11	146–157	154–166	161–184
6	0	149–160	157–170	164–188
6	1	152–164	160–174	168–192
6	2	155–168	164–178	172–197
6	3	158–172	167–182	176–202
6	4	162–176	171–187	181–207

*Source of basic data 1979 Build Study Society of Actuaries and Association of Life Insurance Medical Directors of America 1980.

1983 Metropolitan Height & Weight Tables

Weights at ages 25-59 based on lowest mortality. Weight in pounds according to frame (in indoor clothing weighing 5 lbs. for men and 3 lbs. for women; shoes with 1" heels).

Metropolitan Life ®
AND AFFILIATED COMPANIES

Metropolitan Life Insurance Company
Health and Safety Education Division

1983 METROPOLITAN HEIGHT AND WEIGHT TABLES*

Women

Height Feet	Inches	Small Frame	Medium Frame	Large Frame
4	10	102–111	109–121	118–131
4	11	103–113	111–123	120–134
5	0	104–115	113–126	122–137
5	1	106–118	115–129	125–140
5	2	108–121	118–132	128–143
5	3	111–124	121–135	131–147
5	4	114–127	124–138	134–151
5	5	117–130	127–141	137–155
5	6	120–133	130–144	140–159
5	7	123–136	133–147	143–163
5	8	126–139	136–150	146–167
5	9	129–142	139–153	149–170
5	10	132–145	142–156	152–173
5	11	135–148	145–159	155–176
6	0	138–151	148–162	158–179

*Source of basic data 1979 Build Study Society of Actuaries and Association of Life Insurance Medical Directors of America 1980.

SUGGESTED WEIGHTS FOR ADULTS

Height*	Weight in Pounds +	
	19 to 34 Years	35 Years and Over
5'0"	97–128	108–138
5'1"	101–132	111–143
5'2"	104–137	115–148
5'3"	107–141	119–152
5'4"	111–146	122–157
5'5"	114–150	126–162
5'6"	118–155	130–167
5'7"	121–160	134–172
5'8"	125–164	138–178
5'9"	129–169	142–183
5'10"	132–174	146–188
5'11"	136–179	151–194
6'0"	140–184	155–199
6'1"	144–189	159–205
6'2"	148–195	164–210
6'3"	152–200	168–216
6'4"	156–205	173–222
6'5"	160–211	177–228
6'6"	164–216	182–234

*Without shoes.
†Without clothes.
‡The higher weights in the ranges generally apply to men, who tend to have more muscle and bone; the lower weights more often apply to women, who have less muscle and bone.

Source: Derived from National Research Council, 1989.

Reprinted from *Nutrition and Your Health: Dietary Guidelines for Americans*. Washington, D.C.: U. S. Department of Agriculture/U.S. Department of Health and Human Services, 1990.

II

UNDERSTANDING YOUR "WEIGHT PROBLEM"

What's Your Excuse?

Have you been on a diet since Elvis's discharge from the Army? If so, people (and not very tactful ones at that) are probably asking you, "What? Still trying to lose those few pounds?" And *you're* probably replying with one of the following all-too-familiar lines. Are you simply making just another excuse?

• *"I'm trying to get pregnant right now. What's the point of dieting?"* Although you may have only about 10 pounds to lose, it's nevertheless true that overweight during pregnancy can create or exacerbate certain problems, such as leg cramps and backache. If your doctor suggests weight loss now, take the advice.

• *"I'll lose the weight . . . right after the baby is born."* Of course, you can always diet after delivery. But if you're using your impending motherhood as an excuse to go wild with food *right now,* you're not doing your baby any good and you'll just have more postpregnancy pounds to shed later.

- *"I'll lose weight . . . right after the baby's bar mitzvah."* Uh-huh . . . just don't go near the Viennese table.

- *"Oh, I'm under such pressure at the office! If you worked there, you'd eat, too."* Must job stress be handled with food? Isn't it possible to chew gum/drink mineral water/take a work break and stretch or chat with your coworkers instead? If the job is truly awful, perhaps it's time to get the résumé in order.

- *"I know I should lose a few pounds, but Sid loves me just the way I am."* Maybe he does, and maybe he doesn't. But the *real* question is: How do *you* feel about it?

- *"Tomorrow we leave on our cruise."* True, cruises (and other vacations) are often associated with food and lots of it. But can't you have a good time on a vacation without pigging out? Enjoy whatever you want from the menu, in reasonable quantities, and aim to *maintain* your weight until you return home. Then you won't have set your diet back— *and* you'll still have fond memories of your trip.

- *"I'd like to see you stick to a diet while dealing with building contractors/ shopping with a teenager/ living with Sid!"* All anxiety-producing, to be sure. But, again, food need *not* be the way you automatically handle stress. (See page 100 for specific tips on stress management.)

- *"What's a measly 10 pounds? I can lose it anytime!"* So why *haven't* you? If you can't start today, maybe you never will.

- *"I'll never be thin. Why bother?"* Might this be a self-fulfilling prophesy—you can't succeed simply because you predict you can't? Why not give yourself a *chance* to accomplish your goal and see what happens?

• *"All the guys in my family are fat."* Maybe so, but why not be the svelte exception to the rule?

• *"Restaurant owners (or chefs or housewives or construction workers, etc.,) always have weight problems."* Is that actually true? Have you looked around lately? Have you *never* seen a thin chef or housewife?

• *"I can't lose weight because of the kids and their snacks/ my mah-jongg partners and their bridge mix/ the Girl Scouts and their cookies/ the deli-counter man and his free cheese squares. . . ."* What's next? Blaming Blinky for making you open his bag of Cat Chow?

However you feel about your excuses, they *do* serve a function: They buy you time. Excuse-making keeps you in a holding pattern. You don't *really* have to take any action to change the unpleasant situation you're now in as long as you have a "reason" for remaining there. When you make excuses to others about your weight, you seem aware—you *know* you've got a few pounds to lose—and your "explanation" lets them know you're "taking care of it," that you've got the problem well in hand.

But you don't. You're just kidding people. Worst of all, you're kidding yourself. It's closing your eyes to the task before you and to its level of difficulty. And by refusing to admit honestly that it's tough—and losing weight, however little you may have to lose, *is* tough—you are turning your back on your responsibility for making it happen. After all, eating *is* one of the very few things in your life you can control. You have the power to decide what does—or doesn't—go in your mouth.

Still, the fact is, no one really *cares* if you lose the 10 pounds or not—no one but *you*. Maybe you really *don't* want to deal with dieting right now but are having a hard time admitting it to yourself. That's okay; that decision is as valid as the one to lose the weight.

As for the reactions of others, people who don't much like you now aren't going to start loving you if you drop 10 pounds, nor will that weight loss get you a raise, or make your children more obedient or your father-in-law less crotchety. Weighing 10 pounds less *may* leave you feeling a bit better about yourself, and it may enhance your self-confidence, and it may get you into that fuchsia dress again. And if those things are important to you, fine. But to attempt to "save face" with your family, friends, and acquaintances by cooking up excuses for your weight is senseless. The alibis are foolish, and they only make you look silly, indecisive, and weak.

So drop them. And get on with whatever you decide to do about your weight. Even if you decide to do nothing.

The Secret Reasons
You Stay 10 Pounds Heavier

If being 10 pounds overweight is a relatively new phenomenon for you, then the explanation for the weight gain is probably pretty obvious to you and the remedy is equally clear-cut: less food and more exercise. Some highly frustrated dieters, though, hover just above their ideal weight for months or even *years,* for subtle reasons they're unaware of. If you're one such dieter, then hanging on to your few extra pounds is no doubt a cover-up for other issues you'd rather not confront.

No one's saying you *must* lose the last 10 pounds. However, if you've made them a focal point in your life, it may be because it's simpler to dwell on dieting matters than on other, more complicated ones. Your weight-loss program—or your decision to do nothing about those last 10 pounds—will be easier to live with once you know the underlying *secret* reasons you remain slightly overweight.

1. *Using weight as a smoke screen for your real problems.* Your small weight problem symbolizes *all* your problems and at the same time gives you an excuse to avoid dealing with them. "Once I get thin, everything else will get resolved," goes the thinking. "I'll be able to go out and find a new mate/a better job/etc. I just can't face it now—I have to lose weight first!" Yet you subconsciously know your troubles won't automatically disappear, whether you weigh 135 or 125, and *that* realization is even scarier—and so you hang on to your 10 extra pounds.

2. *Fear of vulnerability and "exposure."* People who've lost even a small amount of weight often experience real anxiety about themselves and their "new body." A part of you is now gone, and although it's a part you insist you didn't want, you can't help but feel different. Some say they feel "smaller" or "less powerful" or "exposed." In any case, you're not the same person you were, which can be frightening, and so you'll do anything—such as hold on to 10 extra pounds forever—to avoid those feelings of vulnerability.

3. *Fear of failure.* "Why should I believe I can do it *this* time when I've failed dozens (or even hundreds) of times before?" So you either don't bother to diet (while constantly complaining about your weight) or you "try" to lose weight but without any real commitment. No wonder you never reach your goal. If you expect failure, usually you get it.

4. *Feeling "stuck."* You're discouraged. You simply can't conceive of looking good or better ("I've always been a little overweight, and I probably always will"), and that belief keeps you from taking the appropriate action. Or the diet seems too hard ("It's just too much effort. Why should I bother?"), or it takes too long (you'd rather have that sundae on Saturday than stick to a diet-and-exercise plan where results take a while to achieve).

5. *Family ties.* Food and eating can be highly symbolic. Some women and men identify strongly with fat people, especially with overweight parents. You love them, you want to be close to them, you want to (perhaps unconsciously) be *just like* them—even if that means sharing their weight problem. Successfully dieting down to your goal weight can seem like a "betrayal" of those you love and the way they are.

In addition, in certain families the loss of weight is associated with illness. Even today, the notion persists that a chubby child is a healthy child and that if he gets thinner, something is "wrong" with him. You may laugh it off as Old World nonsense, but on a deeper level you may believe it.

6. *Fear of being sexually attracted or attractive.* A lot of people report that as they lose weight, their sexual energy increases. It's almost biological—they actually *feel* more turned on. As a result, if they're not currently in a relationship, or if they're trying to avoid their mate sexually, they may deliberately remain 10 pounds heavier to block these strong sexual urges that might otherwise bubble up to the surface.

Also, if you're steering clear of your mate, you may remain overweight deliberately to keep *him* from getting too turned on by you.

7. *Perfectionism.* You're someone who's never satisfied with. *any* aspect of your life—or yourself. *Everything* about you, you believe, needs fixing. Maintaining a small weight problem is simply another way for you to feel less than perfect; your body is just something else for you to keep working on and improving. Taken to an extreme, this obsession with perfection can lead to the eating disorders bulimia and anorexia.

8. *You'd rather eat than be thinner.* Ultimately you believe that being a bit slimmer and all that goes into maintaining that slightly lower weight isn't worth it. Understand that within reason *there's nothing wrong with deliberately remaining heavier*—as long as you're willing to live with the consequences and can stop kidding yourself about your "desire" to be 10 pounds slimmer.

Some of these situations may date to your earliest years and may involve a childhood trauma of some kind. If you tend to "handle" your personal issues by using food, *you've dealt with your difficulties very well.* Assuming you basically feel fine, eat decently, exercise a bit, and are only 10 or so pounds overweight, then *your eating problem is not that severe.*

Of course, if you're worried about your tendency to use food to cope with your emotional problems, you might feel the need to seek professional help. Certainly, if you can afford it, that option is available to you. However, if all you've had is a small weight problem, your situation seems very manageable. For whatever reason, food has become your drug of choice, and while it *would* be nicer if that "drug" were something positive like walking or bike riding, you probably don't have to worry as much as you think.

Understanding your weight problem involves not only getting in touch with your emotions and belief system but also with your *body* and how it feels. Imagine how it would be if you were 10 pounds thinner—really try to *feel* it in your body. Once you do this exercise a few times you may, to your surprise, discover that you're not truly ready to lose weight right now. Stop feeling bad about that. It may be more important to keep the weight on than to take the emotional or psychological risks of losing it. When— and if—you're prepared, you'll do it.

If you're afraid you won't succeed but you *have* dieted down to your desired weight in the past, now's the time to remind yourself of that success, to reinforce the idea that you *can* do it again. Remembering how you've changed before can provide the fuel for change you may need today. Aim for *one* simple physical change to prove you're capable of it. Would you like to be more active, for example? If you usually take your car everywhere, start doing some of your errands on foot. Build on that success and walk a bit longer a little more often. When you see a change in one area of your life, it's much easier to make others.

Or . . . you can choose to accept yourself—and your present weight—as you are.

Why It's So Tough to Lose Those Last 10 Pounds (No Matter How Long or How Hard You've Been Dieting)

If over time you've arrived at the sad conclusion that losing 10 pounds and keeping them off is a lot harder than it sounds . . . you're right. As anxious as you are to reach your desired weight and stay there, you may have already discovered that this can be an exercise in futility.

Starting a diet is seldom a problem for most people, and the initial weight loss—a combination of water, protein, glycogen (blood sugar stored in the muscles and liver), and some fat—is always gratifying to see. But reaching your goal ultimately means *losing body fat,* and fat, unfortunately, is precisely what we gain when we gain weight, and is the last thing to go when we lose weight. And when weight loss doesn't occur with the speed and ease we'd all like it to, many impatient dieters are apt to give up.

Yet the situation is far from hopeless. Understanding the physiological reasons for your last-10-pounds diet woes will help you get past many of the hurdles if you do decide to diet—for the very last time.

BATTLING YOUR BODY

Your body is carefully and miraculously designed to keep you healthy and protect you from starvation—and it perceives dieting as gradual starvation. After all, when you diet you are deliberately withholding the body's usual supply of nutrients and energy sources. The body then starts to fight off this potentially dangerous depletion of energy stores by slowing down—and *you* may experience this as a weight-loss slowdown or even a plateau. The closer you are to your ideal weight and the less fat you have to lose, the more your body is going to cling tenaciously to what's already there.

Some experts label this the "set point," the weight at which your body struggles to remain, regardless of the outside pressures on it to change. "It's a push-pull phenomenon," explains nutritionist Judy Marshel. "When you diet, your body is fighting to release the fat while, at the same time, your fat cells are constantly striving to fill themselves up with *more* fat."

YO-YO DIETING

The "yo-yo" dieting syndrome further complicates things. Whenever you *lose* weight, you lose fat and some lean muscle mass; whenever you *regain* weight, you add only fat. So every time you put weight back on, you're changing your body's fat/lean muscle ratio—for the worse. With every subsequent attempt to lose weight, your body must struggle with more fat than it had the last time around. Then, when you don't see the weight come off despite all your genuine efforts, frustration usually—and understandably—sets in. Your what's-the-use? attitude may then lead to overeating and a regain of the lost pounds. Thus the loss/gain/loss/gain cycle begins once more.

Yo-yo dieting—or weight cycling, as it's currently called—can be more than just frustrating; recent research shows it's also potentially dangerous to health. Dr. Kelly D. Brownell, a psychologist and weight specialist at Yale University, published the results of a 32-year study of weight fluctuation in the June 1991 *New England Journal of Medicine*. The risk of heart disease, including death from heart disease, was 25 to 93 percent higher in the group exhibiting the greatest amount of yo-yoing, regardless of how much or how little they weighed at the start. The study also revealed the added health risks to young females—the group most likely to be dieting in the first place—caused by yo-yo dieting. "The pressure in this society to be thin at all costs may be exacting a serious toll," Dr. Brownell concluded.

While his study is considered controversial and is not universally sanctioned within the professional nutrition/weight-loss community, most experts agree that weight cycling isn't good.

Perhaps the biggest problem associated with it is the way it affects dieters psychologically. "It dates back to your very first diet," says Dr. Xavier Pi-Sunyer, director of endocrinology, diabetes, and nutrition at St. Luke's-Roosevelt Hospital Center, at Columbia University in New York City. "Most dieting problems are the psychological ones, the result of continuously trying and failing. That may be the biggest one you'll need to tackle."

FROM OBESITY TO THE WEIGHT-LOSS FINISH LINE

The 10-pounds-overweight dieter who's been losing/gaining/losing a small amount of weight for years has one type of problem. But the 10-pounds-overweight dieter who's successfully lost a *lot* of weight and is now nearing the diet finish line has a different dilemma. It has to do with the way the weight problem first began.

As a person gets heavier, the more fat accumulates in his fat cells, filling them up from the usual 0.5 microgram of fat per fat cell to their capacity of 1.0 microgram of fat per fat cell. If the person gets any heavier at that point, the existing fat cells will be unable to accommodate the excess fat, and so the body will start manufacturing *more* fat cells—extra cells you can *never* get rid of, no matter how hard you diet. What you'll accomplish if you *do* try to lose weight now will be to empty the fat out of the fat cells below their "normal" size, which your body will interpret as a signal that it's being undernourished. This situation make you hungrier and drives you to eat more, so the body tends to "escape" from the diet it's on—and regain weight.

According to Dr. Pi-Sunyer, that's why very heavy dieters with these extra fat cells "have the hardest time of all returning to their normal weight—and it's probably unrealistic for them to even try." He believes such a person should forget about dropping the last 10 pounds. "If someone went, say, from 150 to 300 pounds, she's better off trying to get down to about 175 than to her original 150."

BORN TO BE BIG

Another possible problem: You may be genetically predisposed to overweight. It's been shown repeatedly that if one of your parents is overweight, the likelihood of your being overweight increases by 40 percent; if both parents are overweight, your own chances are 80 percent greater. By inheriting your parent's extra number of (or larger-than-normal) fat cells, you become more vulnerable to a weight problem than someone with normal-weight parents.

Women dieters are also at a slight disadvantage compared with men. Women usually have more body fat than men, and that additional body fat means their bodies metabolize food less efficiently than men.

Body size is another factor in weight loss. Because women tend to be physically smaller than men, women require fewer calories and a higher level of activity just to maintain their weight. Furthermore, if you're short and small-framed, you'll most likely need to consume fewer calories to lose or maintain your weight than your larger sisters and brothers.

THE ADULT DIETER

Losing the last 10 pounds is a challenge when you attempt to do it for the first time during middle age or later. That's because the older dieter generally must take in fewer calories than the younger dieter to accomplish a weight loss. Blame it on a slowing metabolism. Metabolic rate decreases by approximately 2 to 3 percent per decade, which means that your typical intake may now be *adding* pounds.

What's more, you may never have had even to *think* about dieting until recently. As a result, you might be having a tough time getting into the groove of counting calories and grams of fat and increasing your exercise. Change never comes easily, especially when you're older and when it involves something you've been doing all your life, such as eating.

OTHER LAST-10-POUNDS DILEMMAS

You may have a slight, chronic weight problem that's directly related to a particular medical condition and/or the medication you take for it. For example, corticosteroids, used to treat rheumatoid arthritis, tend to cause water retention and stimulate the appetite. Clearly, as long as your condition persists, you're going to have an uphill battle trying to shed those last 10 pounds. Consult with your doctor to see (1) if she believes dieting is even a good idea for someone with your condition, and (2) if she can recommend a strategy to help produce the desired weight loss.

You must also look at your few extra pounds within the context

of your current life-style. For many people, eating and drinking—
in restaurants, at the homes of friends and business associates,
while traveling—are major social and business events. This is not
to say that you can't control your intake in these situations; of
course you can. However, it may be substantially more difficult
for you than if you're someone who basically eats simply
prepared meals at home. The struggle to maintain a 10-pounds-
lower weight, when dining out is such an integral part of your
work and leisure time, may honestly not be worth it.

THE FRUSTRATING WEIGHT-LOSS PLATEAU

Usually at or close to the last-10-pounds mark, many dieters hit
a plateau. At that point it seems, no matter how diligent your
dieting efforts, you can't get the needle on the scale to budge, for
days or even weeks. "We don't know why it happens," admits
Dr. Pi-Sunyer. "It might be fluid shifts, a redistribution of the
sodium and potassium in the body, or a variety of other reasons."

Naturally, it's frustrating when this occurs, but you know what
you have to do: Stick to your diet and step up your activity level.
If you become more energetic for a while, that will usually get
you past the plateaus.

AND NOW FOR SOME GOOD NEWS. . . .

The weight-loss picture isn't nearly as bleak as this chapter may
suggest. Any highly motivated dieter determined to see her
weight loss to completion and beyond, regardless of her present
circumstances, can do well. John Foreyt, Ph.D., director of the

Nutrition Research Clinic at Houston's Baylor College of Medicine, insists that weight loss is within *everyone's* control. "People use genetics as an excuse for their weight, but the bottom line is *life-style modification*. My parents' genes don't determine how much I'm going to eat tonight or how much I'm going to exercise tomorrow—*I* do."

Feeding Your Soul, Not Your Stomach

What does food represent to you? If you've been struggling with the last 10 pounds for a while now, it's likely food means more to you than just getting your three squares a day. Chances are your favorite snacks have become substitutes for other important elements you believe are missing from your life.

Think about it: What are you *really* hungry for when you polish off that extra–jumbo bag of peanut M&Ms or devour that third slice of pie? Forget, for a moment, what you're eating; the real question is, what's eating *you*? What do you want? A good, loving relationship? Relief from some of the daily pressures? A more fulfilling job? A vacation? A new wardrobe? A baby? A dog?

The recent movie *Eating* touched a lot of nerves in many women as it explored the true significance of food in the lives of some three dozen female characters. As they talked about the intense joys and pains associated with the not-so-simple act of eating, many of the actresses were effectively able to ad-lib their lines, so closely could they relate to the film's subject matter. And it was no accident that nearly every woman cast by director Henry Jaglom was thin (some were even underweight), thus proving you can maintain a reasonable weight and have a good figure and *still* be hung up about food.

Long after the movie opened, magazine articles, talk-show hosts, and women huddled around the office coffee wagon were still dissecting its on-target characterizations and quoting such priceless lines as:

- "Eating is erotic. It's safe sex. I mean, it's the safest sex you can have!"

- "Some girls have husbands and boyfriends and lovers and employers and houses, and I have rye bread and cream cheese."

- "I think I'm still looking for a man who could excite me as much as a baked potato!"

- "Food is the only thing that will comfort me and love me and be good to me 24 hours a day."

If you haven't done a thorough exploration of what your love/hate relationship with food really means, do it now. Pay attention to all the precious time you spend in recreational eating—that is, eating when you're not really hungry—as well as in activities related to dieting—exercising, daily (or more frequent) weigh-ins, trying every new diet, worrying about how "fat" you are, fantasizing about how dramatically everything will change 10 pounds from now. That time could be better spent pursuing those things that will make a real difference in your life and in your level of happiness.

Need help in uncovering your real dreams and goals? Jot down the answers to these questions:

1. When I eat knowing I'm not hungry, I would usually rather be_____.

2. The one thing truly missing in my life is_____.

3. I often eat as a way to forget that_____.

4. I generally associate food with_____.

5. I can talk to_____to help me establish my true goals in life.

6. My ideal life a year from now would be (describe in one paragraph or more)_____
_____
_____.

7. One thing I can do today to move closer to that goal is____
_____.

8. One thing I'd like to accomplish within the month is_____
_____.

9. The next time I'm tempted to eat when I know I'm not hungry, I will instead_____
_____.

Moving closer to the realization of your real desires will help you put food in perspective in your life—whether or not that means deciding to lose 10 pounds.

Who Loves Ya, Baby?, or Why You'll
Never Be Thin Until You Like Yourself First

It's difficult for lots of us to talk about love as it applies to ourselves. "Love myself? Of course I do! What's not to love?" comes a typical reply, usually followed by a gale of not very convincing laughter. No one would truly admit that she doesn't love herself, doesn't value herself just as she is, but look around. Self-love is in short supply when it comes to the 10-pounds-overweight dieter.

When we talk about self love, we're not referring to there's-nobody-in-the-world-but-me narcissism, but rather a healthy dose of feeling good about oneself, of feeling worthy of a nice life. Yet the chronic, slightly overweight dieter frequently has a hard time with that concept.

May I relate a story from my own life? I put much of my life on hold for as long as I was 10 or so pounds overweight, acting as though I didn't deserve new clothes until I was thinner, didn't deserve to have a really close relationship with a man, didn't deserve to earn a good living. Why should I? I wasn't perfect! Far from it! Just look at my *weight,* for example. And the longer I remained overweight, even by a few pounds, the farther I pushed my dreams into the future. Sure, there were people I saw who were, like me, a bit overweight, maybe even heavier, who were enjoying some of the things in life I sought. But it had to be a fluke. Fairy tales can come true, it can happen to you, if you wear size 8. . . .

That's what I believed, anyway. But little by little, as more and more nice things came my way, as my circle of terrific friends expanded, I came to realize that equating a good life with a certain body weight was silly. Once I started paying attention, I noticed that I was reaping the rewards of simply being a competent, caring individual. My boss wasn't asking me to get on a scale to justify the raise she gave me. My boyfriend didn't take a tape measure to my hips before buying me a pair of amethyst earrings. My friend-since-forever Ellen wasn't waiting for me to drop a few pounds before throwing me a fabulous surprise birthday party. Life, and a pretty great one at that, was happening all around me while I was still frantically obsessing about calories. All I had to do—to be accepted, to be rewarded, to be loved—was simply to be *me*.

The question then became: If these people loved me just the way I was, why was I having such a hard time loving *myself*? The answer? Maybe I could. I started to give myself a chance to see and appreciate the qualities in myself others seemed to have no trouble acknowledging. My less-than-perfect body was still a bugaboo, but time and again I reminded myself that it didn't have to be an obstacle in attaining those things I wanted. I didn't need to wait until I lost those last 10 pounds anymore. I was fine and lovable just the way I was.

And funny as it sounds, I started becoming my own best friend, an advocate for myself. I could love myself today, even with the extra weight on me. All along, whenever I sought an excuse to feel bad, there I had it: those last 10 pounds. But I didn't want that excuse anymore. I *wanted* mental health, to feel as good about myself as often as possible.

And so that fundamental change in attitude—from self-indifference to self-love—*made it possible for me to shed the weight*. The cycle had at last been broken. I'm certain it couldn't have happened without a major shift in my feelings about my own lovableness. And had I not chosen to diet off the last 10 pounds, I'm convinced that that attitudinal change would also have made it easy for me to live peacefully with the extra weight. I know, because every once in a while a few of those pounds make a return appearance. But even then, there's no cause for me to be full of self-hate or disgust over "letting myself go," something I used to say. A few pounds more or less on the scale can no longer shake my deep-seated confidence in and appreciation for who I am.

Look around you—at the people who love and admire you, at your achievements, at your skills, at the way you've learned how to cope with the difficult periods in your life and emerge the stronger. How can you possibly let them be overshadowed by a small weight problem? If need be, remind yourself daily of all the wonderful things about yourself, so you can look precisely the way you want to look.

Remember that slimming down your body is optional; fattening up your self-love is a must.

III

MAKING THE COMMITMENT

"I was so disgusted with the way I looked, I finally went on a diet" is an oft-heard remark. Looking and feeling heavy, or not being able to fit into your "regular" wardrobe anymore, is usually the crisis point for people, the time when they know they *must* take action and get thin.

But . . . what if you're *already* thin, more or less? Being (or becoming) 10 pounds overweight is generally not sufficiently catastrophic for us to feel Diet Desperation. We are probably still hearing compliments on our appearance every now and then, and still wear *most of* the clothes we've always worn, and there's still that little voice in the back of our head reassuring us, "You can *always* lose the 10 pounds, no problem!"

So the motivation to diet is minimal—and low-level motivation is the kiss of death to any diet. Even if you *do* launch an enthusiastic, full-scale attack against your last 10 pounds, the commitment to your eating-and-exercise program often slides after several weeks (or days!) of panting for some Heath Bar Crunch. It's that lack of *sustained motivation* that keeps people 10 pounds overweight month after month, year after year.

That's why you're strongly urged *not* to attempt to lose your last 10 pounds unless you're really determined to do it this time—and forever. Especially if you've got a small weight problem, the up-and-down weight loss may be more detrimental from a health and psychological standpoint than merely hanging on to the extra pounds.

If you insist you're determined to lose weight, you must first ask yourself: What is driving me to do it? Distinguish between your *external* and *internal motivation*. External motivation comes in the form of an *outside event or pressure*—a wedding or a reunion you'll be attending, or a warning from your mate or doctor to diet. Just keep in mind that once the event has passed or the weight has been lost mainly to satisfy another person, you're going to need *new motivation* to *keep* it off.

Nutritionist Judy Marshel says that her clients with *internal motivation*—who come to her armed with solid reasons of their own for wanting to be thin—tend to lose the weight and permanently keep it off. These are the people who are dieting for *themselves*. They're tired of being "closet eaters," for example, and now want to live and eat like "normal people." Or they would simply like their clothes to fit a bit better. "The very best results," she says, "are among those who don't view this process as a diet but rather a change for the better in their life-style. They know it's a lifetime endeavor, so they generally end up eating foods they like, but in smaller quantities, and not depriving themselves."

A commitment to increased levels of exercise must also be part of the overall change. Those who are motivated to do some sort of exercise on a daily or almost-daily basis also tend to reach their desired weight and *stay* there. And if the exercise you select for yourself is fun (which it should be), it won't be too difficult to find some time for it each day.

However, we all know that despite the finest intentions, motivation does and will flag. So to help you get going and *keep* going, ask yourself the following key questions. Your responses will let you know whether you need to work on strengthening your sense of commitment:

1. Do I value myself enough to do what's necessary to get the results I desire? (The weight loss must ultimately be for *you*, not someone or something else.)_____

2. What is it about myself that has made it hard to reach my goal in the past?_____

3. What am I going to do that's different to try to get past the weight-loss blocks I've encountered in the past?_____
   _____

4. Can I be happy if I lost just *part* of the 10 pounds—say, only five—and more easily maintain that weight? (Perhaps that will provide you with the feeling of accomplishment you seek and is more doable, given your current situation or state of mind.)_____

5. Am I committed enough to take an ongoing, active role in my weight loss? Am I willing to weigh and measure my food? Record all I eat? Aim for daily exercise? Write down my feelings to help me avoid binges?_____
   _____

Remember, don't start this or any other weight loss/weight maintenance program unless you're prepared to:

- give up your guilt over past weight-loss failures
- change your eating/exercise pattern forever
- stay committed to it, whatever else is going on in your life.

IV

HOW TO LOSE
THE LAST 10 POUNDS

The Quick, Quicker, and Quickest Diets

It may seem contradictory to be offering weight-loss diets after having given you so many sound reasons to forget about dieting and live with your last 10 pounds. It really isn't. The decision to diet or not remains yours; my objective is to help you stop *obsessing* about your small amount of excess weight and be more satisfied with your life, whatever your dieting decision. If losing your weight is crucial to your happiness, then I'd like to make things easier by providing some basic eating guidelines.

As you know, dieting is a very personal thing. For some people, speed—within the framework of a sound weight-loss plan—is paramount, even if that means a highly restricted menu. For others, having more to eat and greater food variety are essential, even if *that* means a longer wait for the pounds to drop off. Particularly if you've been a chronic dieter, you know what will—and won't—work for you. So here is a choice of three eating plans that will help you finally rid yourself of those last 10 pounds:

1. *The Last Ten Pounds Quick Diet.* A slow-and-steady plan offering the widest variety of foods yet keeping to approximately 1,500 to 1,600 calories per day. You can expect to lose 10 pounds within about 10 to 12 weeks on this program.

2. *The Last Ten Pounds Quicker Diet.* A more limited program than above, offering about 1,100 to 1,200 healthful calories per day. You can shed your 10 pounds within approximately eight to 10 weeks following this plan.

3. *The Last Ten Pounds Quickest Diet.* The most structured and calorie-restricted of the three plans, for those who want to see fast results and don't want to be tempted by too many food choices. This program of approximately 800 to 900 calories per day should result in a 10-pound weight loss in four to six weeks while still providing a healthy, balanced array of foods.

Consistency in your efforts is crucial if you hope to see results. Promise yourself that you will be consistent in following this program in *all* its phases: eating properly, exercising regularly, and recording your food-related behaviors and feelings. *Do not* begin this weight-loss plan unless you tell yourself—*and mean it*—that you're not going to quit this time, that even if you backslide, you'll return to the program as quickly and guiltlessly as possible. If this is a particularly stressful or difficult period in your life and you can't *seriously commit to a permanent life-style change,* wait until a time when you can.

Of course, you should get your doctor's okay before beginning this or any other weight-loss program. Especially because you're already relatively slim, he may warn you against losing weight, or urge you to adjust your weight-loss expectations. Take his advice.

Armed with your doctor's blessing and your own powerful

resolve to lose those last 10 pounds now and forever, you should first start by examining your current eating habits. In your Last Ten Pounds Success Diary (which begins on page 66 of this book and can be continued in any ordinary notebook), record for one week everything you eat and drink and in what quantities, *without aiming for a weight loss*. Also indicate whether the food was a regular meal or a snack, and how you were feeling at the time. Was something stressful going on—a dinner-table argument with the kids? Was the food "celebrating" some happy event, such as a job promotion? So often, dieters are simply *unaware* of the foods and portions they take in on a daily or weekly basis. But once you see specifically all that you're been eating—in terms of quantity, times of day when eating or snacking occurs, favorite foods, your moods while eating— you'll easily be able to determine which of the three Last Ten Pounds Diets will work best for you.

The three food plans are detailed in the next chapter. First, though, a few words before you embark on your diet:

A WORD ABOUT CALORIES AND FAT

The secret to losing weight is what it always has been since time began: to burn off more calories than are taken in. Mathematically, it's quite logical: Thirty-five hundred calories equal one pound. Eat an extra 3,500 calories and you'll put on a pound; work off 3,500 calories via physical activity and you'll lose a pound.

Simple. Well, sort of. As it happens, not all calories are created equal. The *types* of calories you take in—that is, whether they come from carbohydrates, protein, or fat (along with such other factors as your metabolic rate and your percentage of lean muscle mass vs. body fat)—will affect the speed and consistency of your weight loss. Because calories derived from fats tend to be harder to shed, you'll see that The Last Ten Pounds Diets are all low in fat.

Another reason for dieters to limit fats: You get more food for your calories when you stick to proteins and carbohydrates. For example, 100 calories "buy" you as little as one-third of a fat-packed brownie or as much as several heads of lettuce.

Given the health risks associated with high-fat diets—including heart disease, certain types of cancer, and, of course, obesity—current government nutrition guidelines recommend that no more than about 30 percent of your daily caloric intake come from fat. All three of The Last Ten Pounds Diets conform to these guidelines.

One important note: While dietary fat should be restricted for the reasons mentioned above, it should not be eliminated altogether. Fat is necessary for supplying energy and essential fatty acids, which is why you'll find *some* fat in each of The Last Ten Pounds Diets.

Just remember that because someone like you is *so* close to your goal, and because weight loss is usually harder to achieve the leaner you are, you have to be *particularly* careful about sticking to your calorie and fat limits. Eat just 100 or 200 more calories a day and the few extra pounds will continue to cling to you as hollandaise sauce does to asparagus spears.

A WORD ABOUT THE SCALE

Believe it or not, the bathroom scale can be your friend, and should be visited on a regular basis. It's those people who say they hate the scale and never go near it who ultimately get themselves into trouble.

Of course, if you've decided *not* to lose the last 10 pounds *and* if getting on the scale causes you tremendous anxiety, you can keep an eye on your size by paying attention to the way you look, the way your clothes fit, and how you feel in general. But if you're following one of The Last 10 Pounds Diets, you really need to weigh yourself regularly to see what's going on. You're kidding yourself if you think you can lose weight consistently without consulting the scale. And isn't it about time you stopped kidding yourself?

The flip side to avoiding the scale—that is, weighing yourself daily or even more often—is equally unwise. Body weight fluctuates naturally for a variety of reasons—water loss or retention, medicine intake, and metabolic changes, to name a few—and you may not get an accurate reading if you weigh yourself too frequently. Keep in mind, too, that the scale is only one gauge of your weight "problem." You may register a larger number than the one you'd like to see because, in fact, you've got a high lean-body mass and relatively little body fat (and muscle weighs more than fat). That means you might be in terrific shape yet weigh more than someone of comparable height and frame with more fat on her. (If you wish to determine your exact body-fat composition, most health clubs or hospitals will give you a free or inexpensive body-fat test using an instrument called a caliper.)

What scale fanatics need to remember above all is that while these numbers *are* a good guide, the quality of their diet, their exercise habits, and their overall health are far more important. Get the scale and its role in your life into proper perspective.

Begin your diet by treating yourself to a brand-new, super-accurate scale. (Sometimes people need to spend a bit of money to take a project seriously.) Then plan on weighing yourself in the morning, before you eat, *on the same scale, the same two days each week,* approximately three days apart. I suggest you *not* make Monday one of those days—Mondays usually have negative connotations for dieters. Try Friday or Saturday, which will help keep you psyched during the weekend, and a middle-of-the-week day, such as Tuesday or Wednesday. You will be jotting down these semiweekly readings in your Last Ten Pounds Success Diary.

A WORD ABOUT WATER

Many dieters avoid drinking water because they're afraid it will bloat them and register a weight increase on the scale. Yet not only is that notion false (the body quickly eliminates any water it doesn't use), but also water is crucial to weight loss for a number of reasons.

First, because a woman's body is 55 to 65 percent water and a man's is 65 to 75 percent water, that fluid must be replenished daily to assure good health. This is especially true for someone who's very active or beginning a new exercise program. Second, drinking plenty of water aids digestion and flushes out the system's waste products. And third, drinking six to eight glasses of water daily will help increase the feeling of fullness—and help you stick to your diet. That's why it's wise to have one or two glasses of water before each meal.

If you drink water throughout your weight loss and maintenance periods, you'll see those last 10 pounds come off and stay off.

A FEW MORE WORDS BEFORE YOU BEGIN

• Buy a food scale and *use it,* to help you make certain you're keeping within your limits each day. Once you start your weight-maintenance program, a good calorie-and-fat counter book will come in handy.

• If you choose to follow either The Last Ten Pounds Quick Diet or The Last Ten Pounds Quicker Diet—where you will have menu flexibility—be sure to select from the food list at least one thing you love every day. That will give you something to look forward to, help you avoid feelings of diet deprivation, and keep you motivated.

• If your 10 pounds are concentrated in your hips or thighs, for example, and you expect this diet to slim you in these areas, you may be in for some disappointment. There's no such thing as "spot reduction." However, you *can* improve the appearance of particular areas of your body via firming exercises. See page 152.

• Get rid of your all-or-nothing diet attitude. If you should happen to "blow it," *immediately* return to your food-and-exercise program. Chances are you won't have caused much damage with one binge.

• Be as kind to yourself as possible during this period of weight loss.

• Seek support for your diet wherever you can find it, but most importantly, be your own cheerleader. Write appropriate slogans and affirmations in your Last Ten Pounds Success Diary to help you get through this period *until all the positive things you're doing become habits*.

• As the Nike commercial says, "Just *do* it." Decide that *this* time you'll give up your excuses and see this through to completion.

• Make the commitment to yourself to be consistent. *Consistency is the key to eternal slimness*.

Food Lists and Sample Menus

Following are sample menu plans for each of the three Last Ten Pounds Diets. All offer a variety of foods and should satisfy nutrient requirements in keeping with government dietary standards. Women can safely choose any of the three programs, while men and teenagers should stick to The Last Ten Pounds Quick Diet, containing the most calories. (Teens should also add two extra cups of skim milk per day.)

It is strongly recommended that women who pick The Last Ten Pounds Quickest Diet—the most calorie-restrictive of the three—do so for *one to two weeks only*. By that time you'll probably see that a good chunk of those 10 pounds is gone, especially is you've also increased your exercise. You should then switch to The Last Ten Pounds Quicker Diet, which will provide you with more food and a continued weight loss at a slightly slower rate. If you choose either of these two plans, you should take a daily vitamin-mineral supplement containing up to 100 percent USRDA. (Although both of these diets contain most of the essential nutrients, the supplements are a good insurance policy.)

The menu plans here are designed to be simple, with a minimum of food preparation—and food temptations. Follow one of these plans until you've become grounded in the basics of low-fat, low-calorie meals. By the time you've reached your desired weight, you'll have learned how to shift your menu gradually to include more of your favorites and more sophisticated dishes—both at home and away—without seeing the unwanted pounds return.

The goal in the following three diets is not only to help you lose weight by reducing your caloric and fat intake but also to help you learn to eat healthfully *forever*. It is hoped that for as long as you adhere to these diets, you will gain some good nutrition habits that will enhance your overall health as you maintain your terrific new figure.

FOOD LISTS

PROTEIN

1 oz. lean meat (up to 12 oz. weekly), fish, or poultry

1 egg (up to 4 weekly) or ¼ cup egg substitute

2 oz. cottage, pot or low-fat ricotta cheese

1 oz. low-fat hard cheese (up to 4 oz. weekly), such as American, Swiss, or Cheddar

2 oz. tofu

1 level tbsp. peanut butter

½ cup cooked dried beans or peas

BREADS, CEREALS AND GRAINS

(WHOLE-GRAIN OR ENRICHED)

1 (1-oz.) slice bread

2 slices "lite" bread

1 oz. bagel, roll, pita, or matzoh

½ English muffin

Melba toast (6 rounds or 4 rectangles)

2 rice cakes or 2 (¾-oz.) breadsticks

¾ cup ready-to-eat cereal (not presweetened)

½ cup cooked cereal (not presweetened)

½ cup cooked rice, pasta, buckwheat, bulgar, or grits

STARCHY VEGETABLES
½ small (3-oz.) potato
¼ cup sweet potato
½ cup peas, corn, lima beans, plantain, pumpkin, or winter squash (acorn or pumpkin squash)
½ cup cooked dried beans or peas
½ medium ear corn

VITAMIN A VEGETABLES
Reasonable servings of broccoli, carrots, greens (beet, collard, dandelion, mustard, turnip), leafy green vegetables (chicory, escarole, kale, parsley, spinach, Swiss chard, watercress)

OTHER VEGETABLES
Reasonable servings of asparagus, beets, Brussels sprouts, cauliflower, celery, cucumber, green beans, lettuce, mushrooms, peppers (red and green), summer squash (spaghetti squash or zucchini), tomatoes

VITAMIN C FRUITS
½ small cantaloupe
½ grapefruit
½ cup (4-oz.) grapefruit or orange juice
1 kiwi
½ medium mango
1 medium orange
½ medium papaya
1 large (or 2 small) tangerine
1 cup tomato juice

OTHER FRUITS (NO ADDED SUGAR)
1 medium apple, peach, or nectarine
2 to 3 apricots, prunes, or plums
1 small banana or pear
12 cherries or grapes
⅓ cup grape or prune juice
¼ small honeydew melon
½ cup pineapple
½ pomegranate
2 tbsp. raisins
1 cup watermelon

MILK AND MILK SUBSTITUTES
1 cup (8-oz.) skim milk, low-fat buttermilk, or plain nonfat yogurt
½ cup (4-oz.) evaporated skimmed milk
⅓ cup nonfat dry milk powder

FATS
1 tsp. oil, mayonnaise, margarine
2 tsp. diet margarine, mayonnaise
1 ½ tsp. salad dressing
1 tbsp. low-calorie salad dressing

O-/(OR VERY LOW-) CALORIE BEVERAGES
Black coffee, tea, mineral water, seltzer, diet sodas

YOU MAY HAVE, IN REASONABLE QUANTITIES:
Bouillon, consommé, herbs, spices, and condiments

THE LAST 10 POUNDS QUICK DIET

Approximately 1,500 to 1,600 calories and less than 35 grams fat per day. Consult the food list for foods and serving sizes.

BREAKFAST
1 helping vitamin C fruit
1 helping protein
1 helping bread or cereal
Reasonable amount 0-/(or very low-)
calorie beverage

LUNCH
2 helpings protein
2 helpings bread, grains, or starchy
vegetables
1 helping vitamin A vegetable
Reasonable amount other vegetable
1 helping fruit
Reasonable amount 0-/(or very low-)
calorie beverage

DINNER
3 to 4 helpings protein
2 helpings bread, grains, or starchy
vegetables
1 helping vitamin A vegetable
Reasonable amount other vegetable
1 helping fruit
Reasonable amount 0-/(or very low-)
calorie beverage

SNACK
1 helping fruit

OTHER FOODS TO BE CONSUMED
DAILY, AT ANY TIME
2 helpings milk
3 helpings fat
6 to 8 glasses water

Repeat The Last Ten Pounds Quick Diet each day until you've reached your desired weight.

THE LAST 10 POUNDS QUICKER DIET

Approximately 1,100 to 1,200 calories and less than 30 grams fat per day. Consult the food list for foods and serving sizes.

BREAKFAST
1 helping vitamin C fruit
1 helping protein
1 helping bread or cereal
Reasonable amount O-/(or very low-) calorie beverage

LUNCH
2 helpings protein
2 helpings bread, grains, or starchy vegetables
1 helping vitamin A vegetable
Reasonable amount other vegetable
1 helping fruit
Reasonable amount O-/(or very low-) calorie beverage

DINNER
2 to 3 helpings protein
1 helping bread, grains, or starchy vegetables
1 helping vitamin A vegetable
Reasonable amount other vegetable
1 helping fruit
Reasonable amount O-/(or very low-) calorie beverage

SNACK
1 helping fruit

OTHER FOODS TO BE CONSUMED DAILY, AT ANY TIME
2 helpings milk
2 to 3 helpings fat
6 to 8 glasses water

Repeat The Last 10 Pounds Quicker Diet every day until you've reached your desired weight.

SAMPLE MENU, THE LAST 10 POUNDS QUICK DIET

BREAKFAST
1 cup tomato juice
1 egg, sunny side up, cooked in 1 tsp.
margarine
½ English muffin
1 cup skim milk
Black coffee or tea

LUNCH
2 oz. smoked turkey breast
2 slices rye bread
Lettuce and tomato slices
¼ cup carrot sticks
¼ small honeydew melon
Diet soda

DINNER
4 oz. broiled scallops
½ cup brown rice
½ cup spinach
½ cup green and red bell pepper strips
stir-fried in 1 tsp. vegetable oil
1 oz. dinner roll
1 tsp. margarine
½ medium mango
Black coffee or tea

SNACKS
1 cup plain nonfat yogurt
1 small banana

OTHER
6 to 8 glasses water

SAMPLE MENU, THE LAST 10 POUNDS QUICKER DIET

BREAKFAST
1 kiwi
1 level tbsp. peanut butter, on 2 rice cakes
1 cup skim milk

LUNCH
2 oz. cold chicken slices
one slice whole–wheat bread
½ medium ear corn
1 tsp. margarine
½ cup cucumber spears
two celery stalks
1 medium apple
Mineral water

DINNER
3 oz. veal chop
½ cup fettuccine
Small green salad with 1 tbsp. low-
calorie French dressing
½ cup green beans
½ cup pineapple
Black coffee or tea

SNACKS
12 cherries
1 cup skim milk

OTHER
6 to 8 glasses water

THE LAST 10 POUNDS QUICKEST DIET

Approximately 800 to 900 calories and less than 25 grams fat.
Follow as written.

DAY 1

BREAKFAST
1 medium orange
½ cup cooked oatmeal
1 cup skim milk
Black coffee or tea

LUNCH
1 slice "lite" whole-wheat bread
2 oz. sliced chicken
Lettuce and tomato
1 cup skim milk

DINNER
2 oz. veal chop
½ cup cooked rice
½ cup steamed carrots
Small green salad
1 tbsp. low-calorie Russian dressing
Black coffee or tea

SNACK
1 small pear

OTHER
6 to 8 glasses water

DAY 2

BREAKFAST
1 cup plain nonfat yogurt
1 cup strawberries, sliced
1 oz. bagel, toasted
2 tsp. diet margarine
Herbal tea with lemon

LUNCH
Chickpea salad made with ½ cup chickpeas, diced cucumber, diced tomato, shredded lettuce, 2 tbsp. vinegar
2 rice cakes
12 grapes
1 cup skim milk

DINNER
3 oz. broiled shrimp
1 oz. whole-wheat roll
2 tsp. diet margarine
½ cup steamed broccoli
½ cup steamed cauliflower
Black coffee or tea

SNACK
12 oz. seltzer
1 medium apple

OTHER
6 to 8 glasses water

DAY 3

BREAKFAST
2 oz. low-fat cottage cheese
1 small banana
6 melba toast rounds
½ cup skim milk
Black coffee or tea

LUNCH
1 cup hot or cold soup (e.g., split pea)
10 oyster crackers
Small green salad
1 tbsp. low-calorie ranch dressing
1 serving low-calorie pudding
Mineral water

DINNER
3 oz. turkey
½ small baked potato topped with ¼
    cup plain nonfat yogurt
4 artichoke hearts
½ cup steamed zucchini slices
Black coffee or tea

SNACK
1 medium orange

OTHER
6 to 8 glasses water

DAY 4

BREAKFAST
1 egg or ¼ cup egg substitute, scram-
    bled, made with 1 tsp. diet margarine
½ English muffin
2 tsp. low-calorie jam
Herbal tea

LUNCH
2 oz. water-packed tuna tossed with
    chopped celery, chopped green pepper,
    and 2 tbsp. low-calorie Italian dressing
1 oz. sesame pita
1 cup skim milk
1 medium peach

DINNER
3 oz. broiled red snapper
½ cup rice
1 cup steamed Brussels sprouts
½ cup fresh raspberries
Black coffee or tea

SNACKS
Diet soda
1 cup plain nonfat yogurt

OTHER
6 to 8 glasses water

DAY 5

BREAKFAST
¾ cup cornflakes with 1 cup skim milk
½ cup blueberries
Black coffee or tea

LUNCH
Pasta salad made with 1 cup cooked
  pasta; ¼ cup each steamed broccoli, carrots, and cauliflower; 1
  tsp. grated Parmesan cheese; and 1
  tbsp. low-calorie Italian dressing
½ cup skim milk
2 small tangerines

DINNER
3 oz. lean pot roast
½ small baked potato
½ cup beets
1 cup steamed green beans with 1 tsp.
  diet margarine
Black coffee or tea

SNACK
1 low-calorie frozen fruit bar

OTHER
6 to 8 glasses water

DAY 6

BREAKFAST
½ small cantaloupe
1 small bran muffin with 2 tsp. diet
  margarine
1 cup skim milk

LUNCH
2 oz. low-fat ham
1 slice low-fat Swiss cheese
2 slices "lite" rye bread
Lettuce and tomato
1 small banana
Diet soda

DINNER
3 oz. chicken breast, no skin
½ cup brown rice, mixed with 2 tsp.
  diet margarine
1 cup steamed carrots
Black coffee or tea

SNACK
1 cup plain nonfat yogurt

OTHER
6 to 8 glasses water

DAY 7

BREAKFAST
½ cup orange juice
1 oz. bagel, toasted
2 tsp. diet jam
1 cup skim milk

LUNCH
Chef's salad made with iceberg let-
    tuce, carrots, chopped celery, chopped
    green pepper, 1 small sliced tomato,
    2 oz. sliced turkey, 1 oz. grated low-fat
    Cheddar cheese, topped with 1½ tbsp.
    low-calorie blue–cheese dressing
1 breadstick

1 medium apple
Mineral water

DINNER
3 oz. baked scrod
3 asparagus spears
½ cup corn
1-oz. dinner roll
1 tsp. diet margarine
Black coffee or tea

SNACK
1 cup nonfat fruit–flavored yogurt

OTHER
6 to 8 glasses water

ADDITIONAL TIPS

• Trim meats and fish of visible fat. Remove skin from chicken.
Bake or broil meat, fish, or poultry without added fats or oils.

• Season food with herbs and spices; avoid salt. Not only may
excess salt lead to high blood pressure, but it may also cause
water retention, which impedes weight loss.

• Initially you may want to avoid dining out so you can get a feel
for the diet you've chosen. Stick to restaurants where you know
foods can be prepared according to this menu plan. Later, at other
restaurants, follow the menu plan as closely as possible when

ordering. Ask for broiled or baked meats and fish to be prepared without butter or oils, vegetables steamed instead of sautéed or fried, plain rather than in sauces, etc.

• If, after following the daily menu plan, you find you're hungry, you may have, in reasonable quantities: black coffee or tea, mineral water, seltzer, diet sodas (0 to 4 calories per serving), green salad (without dressing), raw or steamed vegetables, low-calorie fruit gelatin.

Exercise and Losing the Last 10 Pounds

Think about the thin people you know, and you'll probably notice that they tend to be much more active than you. It's no coincidence. There's just no escaping exercise if you want to drop those last 10 pounds and *keep* them off.

To expect to lose weight by eating less without a corresponding increase in exercise is ultimately self-defeating when you're *so* close to your goal weight. Most experts now agree that it's virtually impossible to sustain any weight loss, large or small, if regular aerobic exercise isn't built into the dieter's regime.

Dr. Judith S. Stern, a professor of nutrition and internal medicine at the University of California at Davis, conducted a survey on dieting that proved beyond any doubt that exercise was key to successful *long-term* weight loss. A whopping 90 percent of those successful dieters surveyed—people who kept off 20 pounds for at least a year—had exercised regularly (at least 30 minutes, three times a week) and aerobically.

What exactly is an aerobic exercise? According to Cal Pozo, a fitness therapist and the author of *The Back Book,* it's one that gets your heart rate going at approximately 120 to 140 beats per minute and is *sustained for 25 minutes*. (It might take you two to three minutes to reach that rate, and it should take you another two to three minutes minimum to cool down.) If you're a moderately active woman or man between 25 and 45, this aerobic workout—ideally done three times a week or more—is what is required to begin burning your body fat. (When you diet without accompanying exercise, you may lose pounds but you only burn a minimal amount of body fat, and reduction of fat is vital for sustained weight loss.) Even after your workout is over for the day, your body is *still* reaping the benefits, because aerobic exercise continues to stimulate the fat-burning process while your body is at rest.

Aerobic exercise also counteracts the slowing down of your metabolism that occurs when you eat less, as you are doing now if you're trying to lose your last 10 pounds. If you've experienced any sort of weight-loss plateau, aerobic exercise, done consistently, should help you break through it.

Activity	Calories Burned from One-Hour Exercise (by an average-weight woman)
Cross-country skiing	1300
Racquetball	700
Rowing machine	700
Jogging	600
StairMaster	600
Swimming	600
In-line skating (roller blades)	600
Step-exercise (intense)	600
Tennis (singles)	500
Tennis (doubles)	400
Dancing (fast)	500
Aerobics class (intense)	475
Aerobics class (moderate)	375

Bike-riding (moderate speed)	450
Stationary bike, at 10 mph	400
Walking (briskly)	350
Walking (moderately)	200
Basketball	350
Gardening	350

WHICH ACTIVITY IS RIGHT FOR YOU?

Check with your doctor before beginning any program of vigorous exercise, particularly if you're over 35. Then aim for a minimum of three 30-minute aerobic sessions per week, more if you can manage. Pick the activity you like and *stick with it*! No more excuses for giving up because you *hate* to exercise—there's *got* to be something from this list you enjoy, or have always wanted to try.

Just remember that if you're not consistent about your exercise program, you'll have a much harder time keeping off the last 10 pounds—or prevent them from turning into 20. As weight-loss expert Dr. Kelly D. Brownell says, "The key question is: Will you be doing this exercise a year from now?" If you can't honestly say "yes," choose another activity.

TAKE A WALK!

Are you the Queen (or King) of the Couch Potatoes, insisting that you could never work a regular exercise program into your schedule? If so, walking's for you. John J. Duncan, Ph.D., associate director of exercise physiology at Dallas's Institute for Aerobics Research, reports that a regular program based on walking a 12-minute mile (almost the speed of race walking) increases fitness on a level comparable to jogging but without the potential for physical injury.

And dieters will be happy to hear that walking is a great weight-loss booster. Even without a change in your present eating pattern, you could still see your last 10 pounds come off in a year if you went on two brisk, hour-long walks each week. But don't let lack of time be an excuse: Even a four-minute walk after dinner can make a difference in your weight and overall fitness level. The positive effects of aerobic exercise are cumulative— several brief-yet-brisk walks per week are still extremely beneficial.

PLANNING FOR SUCCESS

Map out the exercise program you will follow. Don't just tell yourself, "I'll walk briskly for 30 minutes three times a week"; you've also got to plan for those times when you can't or just don't feel like it (and those days *will* come). What if the weather is bad? What if the kids are home from school and you can't leave the house? Have a backup exercise plan. Work out in your basement to an aerobics video, or run around outside with your kids, or make a point of making up the exercise time over the next few days. There'll be unexpected obstacles in your diet-and-exercise program, no matter how good your intentions at the outset, so you might as well plan accordingly by jotting down what you'll do when they occur.

A lot of resistance to exercise comes from hating the way you look in workout duds. It's a nice idea to have exercise clothes you *like* and that help you feel good about yourself. If you're certain that everyone's staring at you as you run around the park or down the highway, realize that they're much more worried about their *own* jiggling flesh than yours.

Once you get into the exercise groove, you may discover—to your horror—that instead of *dropping* pounds, you're actually *putting them on*. The explanation is simple—and ultimately positive. As you begin to exercise more, you're developing more muscle mass, and muscle weighs more than fat. So you may not see a weight drop on the scale because at the same time you're losing fat, you're building muscle.

However, don't get discouraged; in time you may see a loss of pounds if you faithfully continue your diet. Even if you *don't* see the precise number you're longing for on the scale, keep exercising. The worst that will happen is your clothes will fit better and you'll be able to eat more without gaining weight.

THE JOYS OF EXERCISE

The pluses of a regular program of exercise are many. Apart from the weight-loss benefits, exercise helps sensitize your body's appetite-control mechanism, so you're less apt to eat when you're not hungry; it makes you feel better about yourself by releasing tension and minimizing bad moods; and it enables you to maintain your new, lower weight more easily as you increase the food you eat. Exercise with friends, and it becomes a social event as well.

You may not believe it now, but finding a sport/physical activity you love can really be the start of a wonderful new phase in your life. As exercise becomes more and more woven into the fabric of your daily schedule, it will enable you to escape from the relentless dieting mentality that has kept you 10 pounds overweight for months or years. You'll be able to live, and eat, more like a "normal person" than you ever dreamed possible.

The Last 10 Pounds Success Diary

Nothing's better for keeping your eating-and-exercise routine straight than *writing it all down*. Was it *three* slices of bread you had yesterday or only two? Did you walk for 40 minutes or only 25? Once you get used to jotting down these numbers, it will seem less like a chore and more like a way to enable you to focus on other, nonfood-related activities and goals (such as what's going on in the *rest* of your life).

Additionally, keeping a food diary helps you learn your own individual eating patterns—what you enjoy eating and when, which moods trigger a foodfest, which difficult situations you can handle without launching a corn-chip orgy. This detailed information you'll be recording about yourself will be invaluable to your eating/exercise program, helping to keep you motivated and on track.

All of this should take you no more than about five or ten minutes a day. To make it even easier, just start by filling in the spaces provided on the following pages. Do as much of this as you can in the morning to plan your eating, particularly if you have a pretty good idea of what's on the day's menu. Fill in the "My Mood" sections and any food items you can't plan in advance in the evening or the next morning. When you run out of pages, simply use any notebook as a continuous record of your progress.

Day 1

TODAY'S DATE: _____

WEIGHT: _____ (*only* if it's one of your two weigh-in days this week)

BREAKFAST:

TIME: _____

MY FOOD: (include all foods and amounts) _____
_____
_____

MY MOOD: _____
_____

LUNCH:
TIME: _____
MY FOOD: (include all foods and amounts)_____
_____

MY MOOD: _____
_____

DINNER:
TIME: _____
MY FOOD: (include all foods and amounts)_____
_____

MY MOOD: _____
_____

SNACKS:
TIME: _____
MY FOOD: (include all foods and amounts)_____
_____

MY MOOD:_____
_____

NUMBER CUPS WATER: _____

NUMBER MINUTES EXERCISE: _____

TYPE OF EXERCISE: _____

_____

_____

TODAY'S SPECIAL CHALLENGES (stressful periods you anticipate, parties, special dinners, etc., and the specific ways you intend to handle them without overeating):

_____

_____

_____

In addition, you will probably find it helpful to your weight-loss program if you also use these pages to write down your feelings in the following category:

HOW I DID YESTERDAY (your overall reflections on how well you followed the program, periods of stress, how successfully you did or didn't handle them, how you plan to cope better in the future, etc.):

_____

_____

_____

OTHER NOTES TO MYSELF (words of advice and encouragement):

_____

_____

Day 2

TODAY'S DATE: _____

WEIGHT: _____ (*only* if it's one of your two weigh-in days this week)

BREAKFAST:

TIME: _____

MY FOOD: (include all foods and amounts) _____
_____
_____

MY MOOD: _____
_____

LUNCH:
TIME: _____
MY FOOD: (include all foods and amounts)_____

_____

MY MOOD: _____
_____

DINNER:
TIME: _____
MY FOOD: (include all foods and amounts)_____

_____

MY MOOD: _____
_____

SNACKS:
TIME: _____
MY FOOD: (include all foods and amounts)_____

_____

MY MOOD:_____
_____

NUMBER CUPS WATER: _____
NUMBER MINUTES EXERCISE: _____
TYPE OF EXERCISE: _____
_____
_____

TODAY'S SPECIAL CHALLENGES (stressful periods you anticipate, parties, special dinners, etc., and the specific ways you intend to handle them without overeating):
_____
_____
_____

HOW I DID YESTERDAY (your overall reflections on how well you followed the program, periods of stress, how successfully you did or didn't handle them, how you plan to cope better in the future, etc.):
_____
_____
_____

OTHER NOTES TO MYSELF (words of advice and encouragement):
_____
_____

Day 3

TODAY'S DATE: _____

WEIGHT: _____ (*only* if it's one of your two weigh-in days this week)

BREAKFAST:

TIME: _____

MY FOOD: (include all foods and amounts) _____

_____

_____

MY MOOD: _____

_____

LUNCH:
TIME: _____
MY FOOD: (include all foods and amounts)_____

_____

MY MOOD: _____

_____

DINNER:
TIME: _____
MY FOOD: (include all foods and amounts)_____

_____

MY MOOD: _____

_____

SNACKS:
TIME: _____
MY FOOD: (include all foods and amounts)_____

_____

MY MOOD:_____

_____

Day 3 (continued)

NUMBER CUPS WATER: _____
NUMBER MINUTES EXERCISE: _____
TYPE OF EXERCISE: _____

_____

_____

TODAY'S SPECIAL CHALLENGES (stressful periods you anticipate, parties, special dinners, etc., and the specific ways you intend to handle them without overeating):

_____

_____

HOW I DID YESTERDAY (your overall reflections on how well you followed the program, periods of stress, how successfully you did or didn't handle them, how you plan to cope better in the future, etc.):

_____

_____

_____

OTHER NOTES TO MYSELF (words of advice and encouragement):

_____

_____

Day 4

TODAY'S DATE: _____

WEIGHT: _____ (*only* if it's one of your two weigh-in days this week)

BREAKFAST:

TIME: _____

MY FOOD: (include all foods and amounts) _____
_____
_____

MY MOOD: _____
_____

LUNCH:
TIME: _____
MY FOOD: (include all foods and amounts)_____
_____

MY MOOD: _____
_____

DINNER:
TIME: _____
MY FOOD: (include all foods and amounts)_____
_____

MY MOOD: _____
_____

SNACKS:
TIME: _____
MY FOOD: (include all foods and amounts)_____
_____

MY MOOD:_____
_____

NUMBER CUPS WATER: _____

NUMBER MINUTES EXERCISE: _____

TYPE OF EXERCISE: _____

_____

_____

TODAY'S SPECIAL CHALLENGES (stressful periods you anticipate, parties, special dinners, etc., and the specific ways you intend to handle them without overeating):

_____

_____

_____

HOW I DID YESTERDAY (your overall reflections on how well you followed the program, periods of stress, how successfully you did or didn't handle them, how you plan to cope better in the future, etc.):

_____

_____

_____

OTHER NOTES TO MYSELF (words of advice and encouragement):

_____

_____

Day 5

TODAY'S DATE: _____

WEIGHT: _____ (*only* if it's one of your two weigh-in days this week)

BREAKFAST:

TIME: _____

MY FOOD: (include all foods and amounts) _____

_____

_____

MY MOOD: _____

_____

LUNCH:
TIME: _____
MY FOOD: (include all foods and amounts)_____

_____

MY MOOD: _____

_____

DINNER:
TIME: _____
MY FOOD: (include all foods and amounts)_____

_____

MY MOOD: _____

_____

SNACKS:
TIME: _____
MY FOOD: (include all foods and amounts)_____

_____

MY MOOD:_____

_____

NUMBER CUPS WATER: _____

NUMBER MINUTES EXERCISE: _____

TYPE OF EXERCISE: _____

_____

_____

TODAY'S SPECIAL CHALLENGES (stressful periods you anticipate, parties, special dinners, etc., and the specific ways you intend to handle them without overeating):

_____

_____

_____

HOW I DID YESTERDAY (your overall reflections on how well you followed the program, periods of stress, how successfully you did or didn't handle them, how you plan to cope better in the future, etc.):

_____

_____

_____

OTHER NOTES TO MYSELF (words of advice and encouragement):

_____

_____

Day 6

TODAY'S DATE: _____

WEIGHT: _____ (*only* if it's one of your two weigh-in days this week)

BREAKFAST:

TIME: _____

MY FOOD: (include all foods and amounts) _____

_____

_____

MY MOOD: _____

_____

LUNCH:
TIME: _____
MY FOOD: (include all foods and amounts)_____

_____

MY MOOD: _____

_____

DINNER:
TIME: _____
MY FOOD: (include all foods and amounts)_____

_____

MY MOOD: _____

_____

SNACKS:
TIME: _____
MY FOOD: (include all foods and amounts)_____

_____

MY MOOD:_____

_____

NUMBER CUPS WATER: _____

NUMBER MINUTES EXERCISE: _____

TYPE OF EXERCISE: _____

_____

_____

TODAY'S SPECIAL CHALLENGES (stressful periods you anticipate, parties, special dinners, etc., and the specific ways you intend to handle them without overeating):

_____

_____

_____

HOW I DID YESTERDAY (your overall reflections on how well you followed the program, periods of stress, how successfully you did or didn't handle them, how you plan to cope better in the future, etc.):

_____

_____

_____

OTHER NOTES TO MYSELF (words of advice and encouragement):

_____

_____

Day 7

TODAY'S DATE: _____

WEIGHT: _____ (*only* if it's one of your two weigh-in days this week)

BREAKFAST:

TIME: _____

MY FOOD: (include all foods and amounts) _____

_____

_____

MY MOOD: _____

_____

LUNCH:
TIME: _____
MY FOOD: (include all foods and amounts)_____

_____

MY MOOD: _____

_____

DINNER:
TIME: _____
MY FOOD: (include all foods and amounts)_____

_____

MY MOOD: _____

_____

SNACKS:
TIME: _____
MY FOOD: (include all foods and amounts)_____

_____

MY MOOD:_____

_____

NUMBER CUPS WATER: _____
NUMBER MINUTES EXERCISE: _____
TYPE OF EXERCISE: _____

_____

_____

TODAY'S SPECIAL CHALLENGES (stressful periods you anticipate, parties, special dinners, etc., and the specific ways you intend to handle them without overeating):

_____

_____

_____

HOW I DID YESTERDAY (your overall reflections on how well you followed the program, periods of stress, how successfully you did or didn't handle them, how you plan to cope better in the future, etc.):

_____

_____

_____

OTHER NOTES TO MYSELF (words of advice and encouragement):

_____

_____

Even after you've reached your ideal weight and feel comfortable about your eating and exercise habits, you are strongly urged to continue using a diary during the first weeks or even months of your weight-maintenance period. Once you start increasing your intake of food (as you will when you go from weight loss to weight maintenance), it's crucial to have an ongoing record of your food-related behavior, including your twice-a-week weigh-ins. This will keep you focused and let you know if you need to adjust your eating (or exercise) to maintain your new, lower weight.

The Linda Konner Nondiet Diet

Strict menu plans. Calorie-counting books. Weight-loss groups. Diet foods. High-protein shakes.

They're all terrific, and they all work for some dieters. Like you, I tried each and every one of them at one point or another in my dieting life. Unfortunately, I found that nothing that was overly structured worked for me *in the long term*. As soon as I put myself on a diet, I subconsciously rebelled—and before long returned to my usual eating patterns. For me, the secret to losing and keeping off my last 10 pounds was convincing myself I could do it without "dieting" in the traditional sense. As long as I didn't feel deprived, I was able to keep going until I reached my goal weight and, once there, I maintained it rather easily.

In keeping with this theory, the "diet" I worked out for myself didn't feel like a diet in the strictest sense of the word, and it helped me shed the extra 10 pounds I'd been carrying around for close to two decades. It took approximately 12 weeks to effect a 10-pound weight loss, and it was a pleasant experience (as diets go).

None of this, incidentally, is meant to contradict The Last Ten Pounds Quick/Quicker/Quickest Diets, or their effectiveness in helping you finally drop your excess weight. But I found I was more successful adhering to a less structured diet, and you, too, may have good results with this kind of flexibility. Try them all and see which works best for you.

This program's three components mirror the basic format of The Last Ten Pounds Diets: (1) a food plan, (2) regular exercise, and (3) a food-and-exercise diary. The single biggest difference is that my eating plan was very flexible.

First, I began to keep a diary faithfully. For the first week, I merely jotted down everything I ate in terms of food and quantity *without attempting to lose weight*. During this week, I tried hard to avoid making mental judgments about my eating pattern (although, admittedly, it didn't feel great to write down "entire bag [16 cookies] Pepperidge Farm Milano" or "one pint Ben & Jerry's Reverse Chocolate Chunk 'Light' ice cream").

The second week, I started the actual eating-and-exercise plan. My goal was to continue having the kinds of foods I enjoyed (to avoid feelings of deprivation) but eliminating, temporarily, wildly inappropriate items—such as rich desserts and heavy sauces—and my usual larger-than-life portions. Given my basic understanding of healthful eating, I had a reasonable idea of how to create a food plan that was nutritionally sound, appealing to me, and very flexible.

Thus I would stick to the foods I liked that I also knew were generally good for me, such as the steamed veggies-with-shrimp and brown rice I always ordered in my local Chinese restaurant. Instead of my beloved ice cream, I had ice milk or sherbert (not nearly as yummy, but I knew that, in time, I could occasionally have real ice cream again). Instead of whole-milk cheese and other dairy products, I substituted "lite" versions. In place of two-ounce pita bread for my brown-bag sandwiches, I chose one-ounce pitas. I swapped white wine for spritzers.

In short, I retained most of my favorite foods, but made lower-calorie and lower-fat choices wherever possible. I also cut portion sizes by one-fourth to one-third. Happily, after a few days I stopped missing certain foods and those hefty portions I'd been used to; the lighter, smaller meals became a norm I accepted and even liked. (While I'd always known how difficult it was to break bad habits, I was pleasantly surprised to see how quickly one can form and actually enjoy *good* habits.)

As for the exercise part of my regimen, I'd always played racquetball one or twice a week and walked a good deal every day, but I felt a stepped-up routine was now in order. To this weekly exercise I added 20 minutes of jogging or race walking once or twice a week. It wasn't a major increase, but it *was* aerobic, and it helped to burn extra calories. (Once I reached my goal weight, I resumed my original racquetball-and-walking routine.)

For the first time in my dieting life, I was extremely consistent about recording in my notebook everything I ate and drank, how much I exercised, and my feelings during this closely monitored period of weight loss. These daily jottings have been not only crucial to helping me keep track but also remind me of my daily and weekly accomplishments (which I too often overlooked when I was focused on seeing a particular number on the bathroom scale). The diary also helps me anticipate and plan for food challenges ahead.

To sum up:

• Exchange your favorite high-fat/high-calorie foods for lower-fat/lower-calorie versions.

• Reduce your usual portions by one-fourth to one-third.

• Add 30 to 60 minutes per week of your favorite aerobic exercise to whatever you normally do each week. Or if you don't do anything . . .

• Write everything down in your food-and-exercise diary.

Anticipate only a half-pound to one-pound weight loss per week; anything more than that is gravy (so to speak). Looking here for fast weight loss? Forget it. This may be the *slowest* diet you'll ever be on—but it could be your last.

SAMPLES OF THE LINDA KONNER NONDIET DIET

SEPTEMBER 15

Water: 6 cups
Exercise: ½ hr. racquetball; 20 min. race walking; did errands—walked a *lot*

BREAKFAST
1 tsp. diet margarine
1-oz. bagel
Iced coffee with evaporated skimmed milk

LUNCH
80-cal. roll
40-cal. "lite" cold cuts
1 small tomato
Iced coffee with evaporated skimmed milk

DINNER
2 cups fresh veggies stir-fried in 1 tbsp. oil
4 oz. tofu
1 cup steamed rice
1 cup low-fat ice cream (146 cal.)

SNACKS
Iced tea
Seltzer
Diet Coke

SEPTEMBER 16

Water: 6 cups
Exercise: Walked around for 2 hrs. at outdoor book fair

BREAKFAST
Small bowl Rice Krispies
3 strawberries, sliced
½ cup skim milk
Iced coffee with evaporated skimmed milk

LUNCH
½ small cantaloupe
½ cup cottage cheese
1 rice cake
1 tsp. diet jelly
Iced tea

DINNER
White wine spritzer
Small plate penne with pesto sauce
1 tsp. grated Parmesan
Cappuccino

SNACKS
Diet Coke
1 can sliced zucchini
1 cup low-fat ice cream (146 cal.)
Hot tea

OCTOBER 10

Weight: 139 lbs.
Water: 6 cups
Exercise: ½ hr. racquetball

BREAKFAST
½ cup orange juice
1-oz. bagel
1 tsp. diet margarine
Hot tea

LUNCH
Cold salad of shrimp, snapper, lobster
½ large dinner roll
Steamed veggies
2 fresh figs
Coffee with little cream

DINNER
2 cups veggies stir-fried in 1 tbsp. oil
1 cup brown rice
Low-cal. cranberry juice spritzer

SNACKS
Low-cal. hot cocoa (50 cal.)
1 rice cake with low-cal. jelly

OCTOBER 17

Water: 6 cups
Exercise: 17 min. jog

BREAKFAST
Small bowl oatmeal
1 tbsp. raisins
Coffee with evaporated skimmed milk

LUNCH
1-oz. pita
½ cup crabmeat salad
Slice red pepper
Diet Coke

DINNER
White wine spritzer
½ bowl miso soup
Salad with little dressing
Chicken teriyaki
Bowl white rice

SNACKS
Coffee with Cremora
1 medium orange

NOVEMBER 7

Weight: 136 lbs.
Water: 6 cups
Exercise: ½ hour racquetball

BREAKFAST
1 small bowl cornflakes
½ small banana
½ cup skim milk
Coffee with evaporated skimmed milk

LUNCH
1-oz. pita
35-cal. "lite" cheese
30-cal. "lite" roast beef
Diet soda

DINNER
Large portion Chinese broccoli in
  garlic sauce
1 cup white rice

SNACKS
Coffee with Cremora
Tomato juice
½ Kit Kat bar (110 cal.)
1 cup low-cal. ice cream (146 cal.)

DECEMBER 15

Weight: 132 lbs.
Water: 6 cups
Exercise: ½ hr. racquetball; *lot* of walking around

BREAKFAST
1-oz. bagel
1-oz. low-fat Swiss cheese
Coffee with skim milk

LUNCH
½ chocolate chip muffin
Coffee with half-and-half

DINNER
3 cups veggies stir-fried in 1 tbsp. oil
4 oz. tofu
1 cup brown rice
Iced tea

SNACKS
Coffee with milk
1 cup low-cal. ice cream (146 cal.)

DECEMBER 29

Weight: 135 lbs.

JANUARY 7

Weight: 134 lbs.

FEBRUARY 6

Weight: 133 lbs.

MARCH 30

Weight: 133 lbs.

APRIL 29

Weight: 132 lbs.

MAY 13

Weight: 133 lbs.

Perhaps more difficult for me than actually losing the last 10 pounds was making the conscious decision to maintain my weight in the low to mid-130s—that is, several pounds above 125, the cherished weight of my youth. At first, "settling" for those higher numbers was, to my mind, an admission of defeat, until I realized (1) 132 to 134 pounds was a medically acceptable weight for my height, body, size, and age; (2) my body felt comfortable at that weight; (3) it was much easier for me to maintain 132 than 125 pounds; and (4) I looked fine at the higher weight. I'm no longer interested in the *struggle* that was once so much a part of the weight loss/weight maintenance process; I want to stay at a sane weight without making dieting the focal point of my life. I have—and it feels great.

You may conclude, as I did, that the best diet is *no* diet, that you simply make small, significant changes in your current eating pattern. The advantages? You get to have what you like, your weight will gradually come off, and you'll easily and comfortably adapt to any dining situation.

By being *conscious* of what you consume while continuing to enjoy your favorite foods, you're bound to be a weight-loss winner.

How They Did It: Tips and Tricks from the Famous and Not-So-Famous on How They Lost the Last 10 Pounds

Talk to people who've successfully dropped 10 or so pounds on their own, and you're likely to hear some ingenious methods for how they did it. You may pick up an idea or two from these real-life stories:

ELLEN MESHNICK, 43, ad sales manager
Height: 5'6"
High weight: 140
Low weight: 125

"I have found creative visualization to be a boon to my dieting. When I was in my late 20s, I went with a group of friends to Rio de Janeiro, and in those days I was thin enough to wear a tiny bikini. That's the image I keep in my head—me, in that bikini, walking along the beach and looking great—whenever I'm in a situation where I'm tempted to overeat. For instance, when I'm dining out in a restaurant and there's a basket of bread in front of me, I look at the bread . . . and see myself in Rio, in that bikini. I do that and I never *touch* the bread! Even if you've never gotten to your goal weight, you can still fantasize about the way you *think* you'll look at your ideal weight, and use that as the basis for your creative visualization."

CHRISTIE BRINKLEY, 37, model
Height: 5'9"
Weight: 125

"I try never to eat after 6:00 or 7:00 P.M. I may be hungry, but it doesn't hurt to *dream* about hot fudge sundaes! When I wake up, I'm ready for a decent breakfast—some fruit, maybe a small piece of cheese, and a cup of herbal tea."

RAQUEL WELCH, 51, actress
Height: 5'6"
Weight: 118

"I hate to eat when I'm ravenous; it puts me in a ferocious mood, and then I eat all the bread on the table! So to avoid little hunger attacks, I take along snacks to munch on all day. I pack fruit and rice cakes or a small container of brown rice—just a spoonful keeps the wolf of hunger away from my door."

VICTORIA PRINCIPAL, 42, actress
Height: 5'6"
Weight: 110

"I stay away from anything with the word 'cream' in it: cream cheese, whipped cream, ice cream, cream soups, sour cream. If you mentally think of the word 'cream' as 'fat,', giving it up will be quite easy."

MADONNA, 32, singer/actress
Height: 5'4½"
Weight: 118

"My favorite snack is popcorn, but only the fat-free, air-popped kind. I could eat it by the bushel."

JEANNE NOBLE, 40, housewife
Height: 5'6"
High weight: 160
Low weight: 135

"Whenever my weight starts to inch up, I take one of my smaller-sized outfits—one I'll be able to wear when I'm back at my goal weight—and keep it hanging outside my bedroom closet. That way I can see it every time I wake up, go to bed, and get dressed, and it serves as a tangible reminder of the benefits of reaching my goal.

"I realize that I usually overeat when I'm depressed or agitated or lonely. So I keep a notebook on my kitchen table, and whenever I'm feeling 'hungry'—and I know there's no real reason for it—I pick up a pen and start writing about my feelings. It's nothing formal, just stream-of-consciousness stuff, but it lets me release a lot of my fears and resentments, and soon the 'hunger' passes. Another way to let the feelings pass: Instead of running to the refrigerator, I force myself to leave the kitchen immediately. Usually I'll go down to the basement to do laundry or iron, and I don't come back upstairs until I feel safe! The combination of removing myself from the kitchen and letting time pass helps my food cravings subside, and I feel in control again."

ALLEN PETERSON, 37, driving-school instructor
Height: 5'8"
High weight: 180
Low weight: 165

"I will often eat something like a microwaved sweet potato or two or three rice cakes before going out for dinner. That curbs my appetite so I'm not tempted to overeat in the restaurant. Generally, I've shifted to a diet that's basically high in complex carbohydrates, not only because it's healthy but because it's filling."

MARY McHUGH, 51, free-lance writer
Height: 5'2"
High weight: 116
Low weight: 100

"I used to really love Ben & Jerry's Chocolate Fudge Crunch, which I would eat right out of the carton. But then I learned to substitute no- or low-fat frozen yogurt (chocolate almond is great!). It's true that if you eat too much of that, you'll regain weight, but as an *occasional* snack, frozen yogurt is better than high-fat ice cream.

"It may sound funny, but I believe I've actually talked my body into feeling that this is my proper weight, and somehow it resists getting fatter. I've finally learned what a balanced diet is, and I've stuck to it—and I've never felt better in my life."

PETER FRANCO, 45, magazine editor
Height: 5'8"
High weight: 178
Low weight: 160

"I discovered that once I stopped buying junk food—that 50-cent candy bar, that $1.00 ice cream pop, that $2.99 pint of ice cream—I had money I wouldn't have had if I'd not been dieting.

I decided to spend all this extra cash on different types of treats—CDs, books, presents for my girlfriend. This became an additional motivation for me to keep going on my diet."

EDWARD J. MAZUR, 32, high-school teacher
Height: 5'11"
High weight: 187
Low weight: 175

"I keep a food journal. Actually, I use a pocket calendar and record a 'food accomplishment' every day. One day it might be 'Today I turned down Dan's offer to taste his Wild Maine Blueberry ice cream cone,' or 'I didn't touch the chocolates in the box Pauline left out on her coffee table' or 'I walked right past the cheese samples at Hickory Farms.' Every now and then I look over my entries, and I think about how much weight I would've gained had I *not* made these decisions and had not written them down. I've been keeping this journal for two years and it's given me a tremendous sense of accomplishment."

JANE ROSENBERG, 35, baker/caterer
Height: 5'9"
High weight: 153
Low weight: 142

"I gained weight after each of my pregnancies, and another four to five pounds after I quit smoking. I eventually lost my weight by learning to 'bank' my calories. I try to forgo tempting things for as long as I can all day, which means my calorie intake up through late afternoon is minimal. That way I can have some cookies at or after dinner and not feel like a criminal. It may not help you lose weight to eat those cookies, but at least you probably won't gain if you don't overdo it during the rest of the day."

DOLLY PARTON, 46, singer
Height: 5'
Weight: 125

"To lose my weight, I gave myself permission to eat whatever I wanted, but in small portions. For example, at restaurants, I ordered lots of side dishes, but only ate a tiny bit of each. Another tip: When you crave some treat, have it—but only one bite."

ELIZABETH TAYLOR, 59, actress
Height: 5'6"
High weight: 180
Low weight: 125

"A good way to withstand temptation is by waiting it out. When you wait five minutes before having something you crave, and you see you haven't dissolved into a puddle of shakes, you can say, 'Well, I won't have it now; maybe I'll have it tonight.' Immediate gratification is for babies."

CHER, 45, singer/actress
Height: 5'8½"
Weight: 110

"I usually do 40 minutes on my treadmill, which is three walking miles, and about five miles on the stationary bike. Then I have different exercise classes and I have a workout with weights. I vary everything—I don't like doing the same thing all the time."

ART LINKLETTER, 79, TV personality

"I try not to deprive myself of 'goodies' I enjoy. So I order scrumptious desserts several times a week—and then eat only two or three good-sized bites. That's all I permit myself, but it's fun, like cheating a *little*."

RICHARD SIMMONS, 43, diet guru
Height: 5'8"
High weight: 248
Low weight: 145

"You have to get to the point where you like yourself better than food. You have to plan to take 30 to 60 minutes daily to exercise and to clean up your rotten, childish eating habits. Only then can you find peace of mind."

PAUL JONAS, 42, photographer
Height: 5'9"
High weight: 160
Low weight: 145

"I've taught myself to break the late-night-snack habit, as well as conquer the cravings I still get. I had developed a habit of eating at night—say, having an 11:00 P.M. snack—and even after I stopped, my body still craved the snack. So I tell myself that I know I had plenty of food for dinner (which is usually true) and that I can go without the snack I desperately want. The fact that I invariably wake up the next morning without any hunger pangs proves that my so-called hunger of the night before was just a *desire* for food and that I could get through without it."

MEME BLACK, 50, journalist
Height: 5'2½"
High weight: 115
Low weight: 103

"I follow what I call the Psychological Calendar Diet. I don't diet on days when it's psychologically impossible for me to eat wisely—during my menstrual cycle when I crave sweets, or on vacations, or when I'm in a crisis. On those days I allow myself the excesses that I crave, but within reason, such as one fabulous cream puffs for dessert when I'm in England. I don't castigate myself because I know that if I make myself feel guilty, when I return to my normal eating pattern I will go to extremes to compensate for the little bit of overeating. My normal eating habits are moderate and predictable, which is why I've been able to maintain my ideal weight most of my life."

> ANGELA LANSBURY, 66, actress
> *Height:* 5'9"
> *Weight:* 140

"I lost 15 pounds over three months by eating mostly fruits and vegetables and cutting out sugar and red meat. I also walk a lot and ride my bike as much as I can."

> MISS PIGGY

"Never eat more than you can lift."

> MARK TWAIN

"Part of the secret of success in life is to eat what you like and let the food fight it out inside."

> JULIA CHILD, 79, chef
> *Height:* 6'1"
> *Weight:* 161

"Life itself is the proper binge."

> SOPHIA LOREN, 57, actress
> *Height:* 5'8½"
> *Weight:* 125

"Everything you see, I owe to spaghetti."

RICHARD GRAYSON, 40, law-school student
Height: 5'6"
High weight: 160
Low weight: 140

"I used to eat food without being conscious of what I was eating, so I'd eat more than I necessarily wanted to. I would grab a chicken leg or a piece of pastry and eat it on my way out of the house. I've become more food-conscious, which has helped me lose weight. Now I eat as slowly as possible, and when I'm alone I actually cut my food into many small pieces on my plate and eat one forkful or spoonful at a time. For example, the other night I had a slice of cake for dessert, and I cut it into about 20 tiny pieces and ate each piece with my fingers, which made it almost a sensuous experience. Another way I've become more conscious of my eating: I won't eat while reading the newspaper or watching TV. I used to get so involved in the article or program that I didn't realize how much I was eating. Being more aware helps me eat less and enjoy my food more."

PHYLLIS DILLER, 74, comedienne

"It is very easy to stay thin. But to feel good you must exercise; get sufficient sleep; drink no tea, coffee, or soft drinks; smoke no cigarettes; and cultivate the habit of happiness."

V

KEEPING IT UP

Let the Reward Fit the Achievement!

Dieters, even with small amounts to lose, often have a hard time liking themselves because they don't fit their own mental image of physical perfection. So it's no surprise that many of them have trouble simply being *nice* to themselves and that the concept of rewarding themselves can be an alien one. "Why should I give myself a reward?" goes the thinking. "I haven't done anything to deserve it," quickly followed by, "I haven't reached my goal weight yet!" It's an all-or-nothing payoff they've set up for themselves, and when the target is the last 10 pounds, that payoff can seem far off in the future.

But a system of small achievement/small reward is vital to the success of your weight-loss program—*and* makes it more enjoyable. Every major effort, whether it's cleaning a large house, knitting a sweater, completing a college course, or losing a given amount of weight, can—and should—be broken down into small, manageable sections, with a simple but desired reward waiting at the successful conclusion of each section. Life is day-to-day, and so is dieting. Therefore you might as well get the most pleasure and satisfaction out of *every stage* of your weight-loss plan. Stop thinking that the payoff *has* to wait until the very end of the process. It can come gradually and often, as you notice important changes, which may include:

- the improvement of your eating habits
- a diminished interest in junk food
- the increased energy you have as a result of a better diet and more activity
- seeing and feeling your clothes fit better
- the compliments you've been receiving
- a glow in your skin, the result of the water you've been drinking and your improved diet
- a greater zest for living
- an increased interest in sex
- the fun you've discovered in tennis, gardening, running, or whatever physical activity you're now pursuing

If the only thing you had to look forward to after your intense dieting efforts was seeing the needle on the scale go from 138 to 128, you'd be hard pressed to keep going until the end. Instead, why not look at the range of other benefits your dieting is providing, and reward yourself for making those happen as you travel on the road to your goal weight? In fact, if you *don't* plan on rewarding yourself at key stages in your program, you may never make it to the finish line.

Rewarding yourself will come easily and naturally to you once you accept the notion that you deserve it *now,* not when you're a "perfect" size 6. Have you been drinking your six to eight glasses of water daily? Wonderful! Do you head off your binges at the pass by writing down your feelings in a notebook or leaving the kitchen immediately when you sense a feeding frenzy coming on? Great! Have you lost an average of one-half to one pound a week during the past three weeks? Hooray! These are all substantial achievements, and it's high time you took notice of them and rewarded yourself accordingly.

A reward system is easy to set up and will be meaningful to you only if the rewards are given at regular intervals of accomplishment and are items or services that really mean something to you. First, make a list of rewards that will be things you'll truly look forward to having. The list should be fairly long and varied. For example:

- a book by my favorite author
- a long-distance phone call to my best friend in Nevada
- a 90-minute scented bubble bath
- a bouquet of flowers
- a concert ticket
- a manicure
- a massage
- a new cassette tape
- a $25 splurge at the store of my choice
- a new addition to my collection of _____
- a romantic afternoon in the country or at the shore with my mate

Whatever your choice, don't make food your reward. Add to the list as you come up with more and different items that appeal to you. Many of those suggested above cost a few dollars; others involve more of a time expenditure than a financial one. However, chronic dieters often suffer from low self-esteem, which translates into the inability to bestow money or free time on themselves if it's perceived as nonessential or foolish. Believe me, *these rewards are essential* if you are to sustain your motivation to keep your weight-loss program going. The more you learn to treat yourself well and value your accomplishments, the more overall success you'll have.

Some people like the idea of "paying" themselves as a diet incentive (e.g., $10 for each pound lost). If you think this will work for you, fine, but an *immediate* and *tangible* reward—instead of just a heavier piggy bank—is often better.

How do you determine the frequency of the rewards? That, too, is up to you, but they should be based on *specific, measurable* achievements. Here are a few suggestions:

- one reward per pound lost *and kept off*
- one reward for every three 30-minute exercise sessions completed
- one reward for each week you pass up a particular high-calorie/high-fat food favorite (e.g., ice cream or french fries)
- one reward for every seven days that you keep your food diary complete and up-to-date

You get the idea. Many dieters agree that this sort of achievement-and-reward program makes sense but then, for whatever reason, don't use it. They may feel that losing the 10 pounds won't take *that* long and they might as well wait, or the whole thing just isn't necessary. But it is.

Handling Stress

The diet's going well, but . . . every now and then you get stressed out. While keeping stress levels in check is important for everyone, for those with 10 or so pounds to lose, stress can cause havoc for even the most diligent dieter.

What you need is a *lifetime stress plan,* and this may very well be the time when you finally learn the proper way to manage your stress, once and for all, *while* you lost weight. According to

James S. Gordon, M.D., director of the Center for Mind/Body Studies in Washington, D.C., and an expert on stress-related illness, "Any symptom—including a small weight problem—can be used as a vehicle for positive change. Use this process of dieting not only to lose the last 10 pounds but to *change your life*."

Too much to expect, you say? Not really. If you're sincere about finally reaching your goal weight, you'll start tuning in to all those small and big stressors in your life, everything from losing your keys to losing your lover. You can learn to manage your stress in positive ways instead of mindlessly reaching for the Raisinettes—*before* the waistband on your pants gets any tighter.

Following are some strategies for combating stress—and staying slim:

1. *Feel* the stress in your body. Stress produces real physiological symptoms. Your first step is to figure out what they are. Is it a tightening of your gut? Sweatiness? Restlessness? Hunger pangs? Begin to recognize the early signals of your food cravings.

2. Work on your tension spots. Most of us barely have an inkling of where our tension lies. If you've been sitting at the computer for three straight hours, you may get anxious—and unconsciously grab for something sweet or crunchy—when it's simply a case of tense muscles. Deliberately *increase* the tension in your muscles (scrunch your shoulders, for instance), breathe in and out several times, then relax. You'll feel better than if you'd eaten a doughnut you didn't want.

3. Ask yourself: How do I feel emotionally? What's upsetting me? In your Last Ten Pounds Success Diary or in a separate

notebook, write down your feelings, the events and/or people bothering you—whatever is making you tense. How do they relate to your eating patterns?

4. Make the necessary changes. Once you've identified the parts of your life causing you stress, *act*. Is your awful job making you nibble at the office? It may be time for a new job. If your relationship is stressful and you start eating when your husband comes home because it's easier than talking to him, *deal* with that situation. If you don't like something in your life, do something about it—or work on yourself so you can cope better.

5. Eat balanced, nutritious meals. Poor dietary habits can actually *cause* stress, and you've got enough already. Not certain that you're getting adequate nutrition from your meals? Switch to the Last Ten Pounds Quick Diet—a good, basic eating plan for anyone. Minimize your intake of sugar and caffeine, both of which can actually cause tension and anxiety after their initial energy boosts wear off. Also avoid food additives, which can increase feelings of agitation and may ultimately cause you to overeat.

6. Exercise regularly, and especially when you feel stress coming on (or getting worse). It's been shown in study after study that a period of vigorous exercise—even if it's just a brisk, 20-minute walk—is not only physically beneficial but also helps ease worry, anxiety, and tension.

7. Try Yoga or meditation. Low-cost classes are probably available in your area, or rent a videotape. Many people have reported tremendous reductions in their stress level following their Yoga or meditation sessions.

Dressing 10 Pounds Skinnier While You're Losing Weight

We've all had this experience: Someone tells you that you look like you've lost weight when you actually weigh the same or *more* than you did the last time that person saw you. Hmm . . . It's not so bizarre. Chances are it has to do with the outfit you have on that day. Clothes can make you look tubby or terrific, regardless of the number on your bathroom scale.

While you're dieting off your 10 pounds, there are things you can do fashionwise to look slimmer *instantly*. It's all in the cut, color, and style of your wardrobe. Below, two fashion experts offer their suggestions for looking your thinnest *right now:*

WOMEN'S WEAR

This information comes from fashion expert Beryl Meyer, former fashion writer for *Harper's Bazaar* and coauthor of *Style: Developing the Real You.*

COLOR

Color plays a key role in a thinner appearance. Monochromatic (tone-on-tone) dressing creates the illusion of a leaner, lankier figure. That's because wearing one color from shoulder to foot creates a continuous—and slimming—line. As the eye follows that line, your lumps and bumps are pared down, streamlining your shape. If you want a variation on the one-color look, at least aim to keep the colors closely matched or within the same range. Just a subtle difference in tone will make your outfit interesting and still produce that slimming effect.

Deep tones are the most slenderizing, but this doesn't mean you need to limit your wardrobe to solid black. Experiment with other dark shades, such as rich browns and midnight blues, which are just as kind to the 10-pounds-heavier figure as is black.

Where you place the color is just as important as the color itself. Because dark colors minimize, they belong on the heaviest part or parts of your body. So if big thighs are a problem, for instance, your skirt, pants, or the lower part of your dress should be in the darkest tones. Conversely, light or bright colors are magnets for the eye, so you'll want to wear them where you're slimmest, thereby diverting attention away from your extra weight.

Graphic color-blocking on a dress or suit can also create the illusion of a slimmer body. Look for snappy color combinations that "carve" a new, smaller shape. Best: a neutral or bold color bordered in black. From a distance, the dark outline "disappears" the black outline—along with your excess weight.

To ensure a continuous, elongating line of color, match your hose to your skirt or pants and shoes, or go for a slightly darker shade.

PROPORTION

The proportion of your clothes can make you look 10 pounds lighter—*or,* if you're not careful, 10 pounds heavier. The most flattering proportion for the slightly overweight figure is *long* over *lean* (or *long* over *short,* if your legs are great). This translates into a long jacket or other top that falls just past the derrière, worn over a narrow skirt or pants. If your jacket ends too high up on your body, it will bring the eye to the trouble zone—and cutting the line there will make your bottom appear even wider.

The rule is slightly different if you're petite (5'4" or shorter). Look for separates specially designed for petite women, and choose a jacket that's waist- or hip-length for the most flattering—and slimming—style.

SHAPE AND FIT

The shape and fit of your clothes can redefine your figure almost instantly and help make you look pounds lighter. Most slightly overweight women assume that bigger clothes are better for hiding bulges. But the fact is that oversize outfits can actually *add* the illusion of extra weight.

So choose outfits that have at least a *bit* of a waistline— whether or not yours is ideal. A waistline makes you look curvier from shoulder to thigh. Anything that narrows the body—slim-leg pants with a slightly loose fit; tapered legs, such as pants with stirrups; a wrap skirt; a chemise dress with a slightly pegged hem—visually takes off pounds.

If you don't feel comfortable in clothes that are close to the body, wear easy-fitting, flared styles. Swing dresses and coats, as well as trapeze tops, are effective in disguising weight as they skim over your less-than-perfect areas. If you pick a flared jacket, pair it with a slim-lined skirt or pants—again, for that flattering proportion.

PATTERN

Clothing pattern follows the same principle as clothing color: The more eye-catching, the more it should be confined to the best parts of your body. So choose a bold print—a flower pattern, for example, with each image no larger than your fist—and wear it at the slimmest parts of your body to shift the focus there. If you love small prints—tiny dots or checks, for instance—you can wear them, but don't limit them to one spot. Instead, make sure the pattern covers the entire outfit, from shoulder to hemline, for that all-important elongating line. Vertical stripes are obviously the most slimming of all patterns, so choose those often.

Never wear more than three patterns or colors at a time—that busyness only adds the appearance of pounds. Anchor those colors you do wear with the darkest color in the background, covering as much of your body as possible.

FABRIC

Look for fabrics that drape your body easily; avoid those that are either too tight or too bulky. Lightweight wool, cotton, rayon, and crepe are your best bets. Steer clear of anything too stiff—it will make your body look boxy.

DETAILS

Beware of details that might emphasize body flaws and tack on inches to a thick middle, wide hips, or large bottom. Avoid pant cuffs, big flap pockets at the hip—anything that visually cuts your height and subsequently adds width to your frame. And skip wide, elastic waistbands (they balloon out, above and below the waistline) in favor of a waistband that's inset and gives a smoother, trimmer line.

Anything that buttons down the front—be it a cardigan jacket or a coatdress—moves the eye in a vertical line and is flattering as well as slimming.

SPORTSWEAR

After work and on weekends, don't just settle for your baggy old sweatshirt and sweatpants. Not only do they look bulky, but they'll also provide you with absolutely no motivation to get out and move around! Instead, opt for sleek-but-comfy leggings or stirrup pants, which have the built-in stretch of Lycra and the slimming power of spandex (for control similar to that of a girdle but with lots more comfort). These kinds of legwear are better for most women than jeans, which are "heavier"-looking and may actually highlight your bulges. On top, wear a big shirt or slightly oversized sweater. (Again, watch out for excess bulkiness.)

Even if you're 10 pounds overweight, fear not: You can still wear shorts. Just make sure that they end at the *slimmest* part of your leg (usually four inches above or just below the knee). The fabric should drape easily, falling close to—but not tight against—your leg.

As for bathing suits—yes, you can wear them, too—choose wisely. Look for those that have a mix of bold color for the areas of your body you want to play up, plus slimming black or navy for those parts you want to minimize. Consider a sarong-style suit, which is extremely flattering for women with a slight weight problem. Their advantages: The skirt covers the top of the leg (thus disguising unsightly lumps and bumps), and the wrapped waist or hip is both stylish and slenderizing.

Other tips: Try a two-piece suit that you can buy in different sizes for top and bottom; or one of the "slimsuits," such as those created by Carol Wior, designed to shape a slightly overweight body. Just keep in mind that some women have reported that these body-hugging suits feel like a corset, and you may have to decide whether, as *Saturday Night Live*'s Fernando used to say, it's better to look good than to feel good.

ACCESSORIES

Jewelry and other accessories can actually help create the long, slim visual line you seek. Select long chain necklaces that fall midway between your bust and waist and/or long, dangling earrings—both "stretch" and slim your face and overall frame. Avoid tiny earrings or too-delicate jewelry (it'll look lost on you) and thick pearl chokers and other chunky pieces (they'll overwhelm you).

Belts needn't be avoided if you're a few pounds overweight. Just be sure to wear your belt loosely, letting the ends drop slightly on the hip, to further elongate your torso.

Shoes with a contrasting color at the toe, such as Chanel's two-tone classic styles, not only narrow the look of your foot but also draw the eye downward (and away from figure flaws).

UNDERWEAR

Underwear is like a check-in device: When you put it on every day, you instantly get in touch with your body. And the best undergarments are those that not only feel good but also help you look thinner in your clothes. Make sure your bra fits properly and gives your bust the right support—a saggy bra can mean a saggy (and heavy-looking) bustline. You can also buy a bra specifically designed to minimize large busts.

The newest figure-trimmers are "hip slips," sleek, mini-length slips (short enough to wear under short skirts) with the shape-molding power of Lycra. A generation or two removed from old-fashioned girdles, these "slips" smooth and slim bulging hips and saddlebags, making your body look great under clothes.

MENSWEAR

These facts are from Elaine Gross, international men's fashion design and marketing consultant:

FIT

Fit is foremost! If what you're wearing is too tight, you'll look like a stuffed sausage, and if the outfit is too large, it'll make you look dumpy and heavier than you are. (Forget the common belief that bigger clothes are better if you're overweight: They may cover up your problem areas but won't necessarily make *you* look smaller.) The importance of fit also applies to sleeve and pant lengths: Too short and you'll look squeezed in, too long and you'll seem lost in your clothes.

How do you determine proper fit? If you're not confident of your own ability to judge it, shop at reputable menswear or specialty stores and ask the salespeople for their advice. They're usually trained in fit and alterations, so their opinions tend to be sound.

COLOR

It's still true that dark-toned colors make you appear slimmer, but you don't necessarily have to wear *only* black or charcoal gray. Medium and bright colors, in certain circumstances, will also give the illusion of a trimmer body.

The navy blue suit—and particularly navy blue pinstripe—has been called the "power suit" for good reason: Not only does the dark color conceal your few extra pounds, but also the pinstripes elongate the body. Suits in general help to improve the look of your body, because the two matched garments on top and bottom create a longer, more linear silhouette.

Avoid pastels and white or very light-colored suits or jackets and slacks—these colors visually add weight to the body. Medium-range tones, including khaki and light camel, are fine.

Black men and others with dark skin should stick to darker-toned suits.

STYLE

Double-breasted suits and jackets are better than single-breasted styles. That's because men often carry their excess weight in their belly, and the two rows of buttons found on double-breasted jackets shift the focus from the stomach area to the sides of the body.

Wear fewer rather than more layers, which add bulk to the body. Stick to two-piece rather than three-piece suits, for instance.

FABRIC

Stay away from thick, bulky fabrics–tweeds, corduroy, anything with a lofty or hairy surface. Flat but textured fabrics are good alternatives to plain solids—for example, crepes and anything with a vertical line, such as seersucker. And you can't go wrong with those old standby gabardines, flannels, and plain-weave fabrics.

SUITS AND JACKETS

The current trend toward casual, lightly constructed jackets is a blessing for the slightly overweight man. These jackets are generally not fitted at the waist and are often unlined or partially lined—which creates less bulk and allows them to drape softly over the body without molding to it.

The placement of the gorge (the point where the lapel and collar meet) and the buttons can visually slim and lengthen your body. The higher the gorge and the higher the placement of the top button on the jacket, the better.

VESTS

A loose-fitting, casual vest makes a good cover-up for a flabby belly. But avoid vests that are part of a three-piece suit—the extra layers add bulk.

PANTS

Slightly tapered-leg trousers have become the best-selling silhouette during the past few years, and for good reason: They're slim without being too skinny, and their fuller cut at the top, narrowing to the hem, helps disguise big bellies and gives an all-over slim look.

Pleated pants are preferable to plain fronts, because the pleats help camouflage tummy bulges.

Stay away from cuffed pants—the excess fabric at the hem weighs down the silhouette and makes legs look stubby.

Denim jeans are great for slightly overweight men, because they act like a girdle. But don't wear extremely tight or extremely baggy jeans for reasons mentioned earlier; make sure they fit you perfectly.

SHIRTS AND TIES

Shirts that contrast with the rest of your outfit, as well as colorfully patterned ties, help to shift the eye from your problem areas. But when choosing shirts, avoid big, splashy plaids in favor of solids. Exceptions: very small-scale checks, window-pane plaids or stripes. Be extracautious with fitted (tapered) shirts, which have the unfortunate habit of clinging to pot bellies.

Knit shirts, including polo shirts and Ts, are fine if they're not too fitted or made of thin, clingy fabric. Casual shirts worn over pants (not tucked in) are great for concealing any waist-area problems. Don't be afraid to buy these shirts in bold, colorful prints.

Turtlenecks in any color are also fine—they're great for covering up heavy necks and double chins. But as with any knit top, they shouldn't be too fitted.

SWEATERS

Avoid any that are too short or too fitted. Stick to flat, fine-gauge knits as opposed to bulky, heavily textured styles.

COATS

Stay away from styles that are very bulky or have an obvious waistline (e.g., fully belted coats, but back belts are okay). Any color that's not too loud or bright is fine.

SHORTS AND BATHING SUITS

The rule about not wearing too-large or too-long clothes does *not* apply to shorts and bathing suits. Bermuda shorts that hover around the knees are much more flattering than shorter ones. As for swimwear, *please:* No bikinis or body-hugging styles—trunks and boxer styles are best. (Exception: If you're only a pound or two away from your ideal weight, "power-stretch" fabrics with Lycra spandex can flatter your shape by acting as a girdle.)

All the color rules apply to shorts and bathing suits, but if you want to buy bright-colored items, make sure they're full, rich tones and not pale or whitened shades, which will only draw attention to the body flaws you're trying to conceal.

ACCESSORIES

Keep them to a minimum. This is one case where less is truly more. If you wear a pocket square, make sure it's neat and trim, not floppy and oversized.

Suspenders are preferable to belts, which can call attention to your waistline by breaking up the vertical line.

Avoid heavy, clunky, thick-soled shoes—they make your leg and overall silhouette look chunky. Choose dark-colored, slim styles. (Exceptions: walking or running shoes, hiking boots.)

OTHER DRESSING TIPS FOR WOMEN AND MEN

1. Go through your closet and give away everything that makes you look heavy. *You* know which outfits they are: the expensive ones, the impulse-purchase items, and those with sentimental value that just don't flatter you. You're better off without them. With a closetful of garments that make you look as slim as possible, you'll feel better about yourself instantly. If you're game, have a honest-yet-tactful friend come over while you try on different outfits, and let her or him help you decide what should stay and what should go.

2. Love to shop for clothes? Use that as an incentive to keep you motivated to stay on your diet. Plan on buying new items as your rewards.

3. Dress as well as you can as often as you can. No need for the cocktail dress for your trip to the supermarket; a casual but neat outfit will do. The point is that the more you're concerned about your appearance *in general,* the better you'll feel about yourself and the less you'll dwell on your weight.

Makeup and Hair for a Slimmer Face

For many women, the first place their weight loss will show is in their face (darn it). If you're one of those people with a naturally full, round face, you know that it can emphasize overall heaviness. Poor makeup application and certain hairstyles will only compound the problem.

You can give the illusion of a slimmer face with the way you do your makeup and hair. According to Adele Fass-Licata, makeup director at Ashton & Company, a New York City spa and beauty salon, "Proper makeup application is a great way to deflect attention away from your extra few pounds and to your face. When your features are made up beautifully, *that's* what people will see, not your weight."

She shares her makeup and hair tricks:

SHAPING A "SLIMMER" FACE

The key to "sculpting" a more delicate, beautiful face is contouring. Start by applying foundation, which should exactly match the color of your neck, and translucent loose powder, in a tone one or two shades lighter than your foundation. Contouring can help "slim down" wide or fleshy areas of the face, but be very careful: Contour powder that's too dark or badly applied will only make your face look dirty. So choose a shade of contour powder that's flesh-colored, perhaps pinkish brown or soft tan. Then, with a small blusher brush, apply the contour powder along the jawline, making absolutely sure to blend the edges *completely*. (You don't want to look like you have a dark smudge around your jaw.)

Next, brush a bit of the contour powder just in front of your ears and along the temples and the outer sides of the face—a nifty trick for "slimming down" a round face. You can also "create" cheekbones if you can't find yours by applying the powder in the "hollows" of your cheeks, just under the ridge where the cheekbones would be. (You'll find the hollows by pressing with your fingertips under the edges of the cheekbones, right where you feel your molars.) Contouring in these areas will give more structure to your face and take away some of the roundness.

COLOR ME THIN: LIPS AND CHEEKS

If your face is naturally full, dark or bright makeup colors can make you look clownlike and will only "enlarge" the areas where you apply them. Conversely, muted colors make things look smaller. So you're better off using softer shades, but they don't have to be dull; try the in-between color range. Avoid blusher and lipstick colors such as bright reds and fuchsia, bright corals or oranges—they're too garish and not flattering to round cheeks or very full lips. Instead, select brownish pinks, soft fuchsias, soft mauves, dusty pinks, and delicate rose reds. Use a matte or cream lipstick, not the frosted kind, which make things look rounder and would therefore accentuate the fullness of your lips.

Lips should first be cleanly defined with a lip pencil. Then, after you've applied your lipstick, make sure it overlaps the lip liner outline. (Lip liner should never be visible.)

COLOR ME THIN: EYES

The same color rules for lips and cheeks apply to eye makeup, so stick to the more muted shades. That means dusty teals rather than bright turquoises; soft mauve, eggplant, or plum rather than bright purple; dusty pink instead of bright pink.

Choose a light, medium, and deep shade of the same basic color. Apply the light shade as an underbase, all over the eyelid; the medium color along the lashes and extending upward, almost to the eyebrow; and the darkest shade just in the outer corner of the eye. Almond-shaped eyes "slim" the best. Aim for a soft, rounded shape that comes up and out slightly at the outer corner. Avoid an angular eye shape—it's too extreme-looking for most women. If you have puffy eyelids, bring the darkest color into the creaseline, to help reduce the puffiness.

Unless you're deliberately going for a retro 1960s look, skip the hard-edge line you get when using liquid eyeliner. Opt for pencil liner above the lashes, and soften and slightly smudge the line at the edges. Then apply another soft line using the pencil or some eyeshadow along the lower lashes, to "open up" your eyes and help make your cheeks look less full. Add plenty of mascara—it makes eyes sparkle.

When you're done applying your eye makeup color, it should resemble an Impressionist painting, with the shades all flowing together; there should be no hard edges. If you detect distinct blocks of color on your eyes, go back and blend some more.

HAIR

If you're a bit heavy, with a roundish face, you'll want to frame it softly—and if your hair is too pulled back, it will make you look "all face." So avoid extreme styles, such as stick-straight hair and geometric cuts, which will make you look hard and emphasize the fullness of your face. Ideally, your hair should be slightly curled and layered. Go for some height—that will make your face appear a bit smaller, and your whole silhouette will, in turn, look smaller.

If you wear bangs, they should also be soft, slightly feathery, and a bit asymmetrical, with some forehead showing through to elongate the face. Avoid flat-against-the-forehead bangs, which cut the face in half and make it look fuller.

EYEGLASSES

Wear eyeglasses? The shape of your frames can help "narrow" your face as much as makeup and hair can. Slightly wider frames can make a full face appear slimmer. Avoid frames that fall within the borders of your face; they'll only add width.

VI

WEIGHT MAINTENANCE, OR HOW TO KEEP IT FROM BECOMING THE LAST 11 POUNDS

If you've just concluded one of the Last Ten Pounds Diets and have finally reached your goal weight, hooray for you! You're now ready for maintenance.

It's impossible to stress sufficiently how important it is for you to work as diligently to *maintain* your weight as you did to lose it. As we've already discussed in this book, weight yo-yoing (or weight cycling) is not only frustrating but also potentially dangerous to your health. This is particularly true if you've spent the past several weeks or months conscientiously monitoring your eating and exercise to lose weight; the last thing you want now is to undo all your good work and see the pounds pile back on. (And you already might know how easily that happens.)

Think of maintenance as a *continuation* of the beneficial phase you've just experienced, rather than the *end of a diet,* and chances are good you'll be successful. That thought will help you deal with the harsh reality of weight maintenance: You're never *completely* off the hook. You *can't* simply return to the old eating and nonexercising behaviors that got you overweight in the first place. Sensible eating habits and almost-daily (or daily) exercise *must* become part of your life-style if you're going to stabilize your 10-pounds-lighter body weight.

Happily, maintenance has a big plus: You get to eat more than during the dieting phase, including those favorites you may have temporarily given up. Foodwise there's nothing off-limits to you now, as long as you make an effort to continue to eat a basically healthy, balanced diet, with reasonably sized portions. The goodies you've missed can again be yours—*if* you want them (don't be surprised if you've actually lost your taste for high-fat ice cream and greasy fried foods) and *if* you eat them in moderation. Now's the time to sample the brand-new, ever-expanding varieties of low-calorie/low-fat foods (again, in moderation). There's practically no food category that doesn't boast an array of "lite" versions. If you *must* control your weight, this is the most wonderful time in culinary history to be doing it. Enjoy it!

How much more food should you be consuming now? Start by increasing your daily intake by about 100 calories, concentrating on breads and grains, fruits and vegetables. However, a daily or weekly splurge on a favorite 100-or-so-calorie food item is fine if it'll boost your commitment to the rest of your eating program. Invest in a calorie-and-fat counter book to help you make wise food selections. And if you see that your eating is getting a bit out of hand, return to the Last Ten Pounds Quick Diet for as long as you need to, to get you back on track.

You've probably gotten used to a stepped-up exercise regime by this time, which will hold you in excellent stead as you now strive to keep your weight stable. Study after study proves that the most successful *long-term* weight maintainers exercise aerobically every day for a minimum of 30 minutes, or fairly close to it.

Continue to monitor your weight with your twice-a-week weigh-ins, and adjust your calorie intake accordingly. If you find you're still losing weight, add another 100 calories or so a day; if you're gaining weight, return to the Last 10 Pounds Quick Diet. And if your weight remains within the same one-to two-pound range of your goal, week after week—perfect!

Summary

1. Add 100 or so calories per day.

2. Exercise aerobically 30 minutes per day, as many days a week as possible.

3. Continue to record foods and feelings in the Last Ten Pounds Success Diary every day for at least two to four weeks.

4. Weigh in twice a week.

5. Add or subtract calories as necessary.

6. Plan on maintaining this weight forever.

The Last 10 Pounds Pitfalls

Every dieter has pitfalls to guard against during weight-loss maintenance. Here's what you need to watch out for. There's no need to worry if these situations crop up—as long as you know how to cope.

Pitfall: "I've gained back a little weight—and I've been so good!"
Solution: Occasional small gains are perfectly normal. If you're a woman, it could be temporary water weight (are you expecting your period?), and it will probably be gone by your next weigh-in. Otherwise, ask yourself: Have I been *very* consistent regarding my diet, exercise, and diary-keeping? If not, start now! Be scrupulous about *everything* you eat, so you're aware of those little extra calories that have been sneaking onto your spoon. Step up your vigorous exercise by at least 30 minutes a week. Keep going, and soon you'll be back to the weight you want.

Pitfall: "Help! My mate is trying to sabotage me!"
Solution: Diet saboteurs are particularly dangerous when you're at your goal weight. Now, more than ever, you're likely to hear, "C'mon! One little piece of cake won't kill you!" True—but the decision to eat or not to eat should be yours. Watch out for those "helpful" family members or other fellow diners who may—for reasons that are psychologically healthy or otherwise—wish to steer you toward *their* way of eating. No one knows better that you what you need right now. Thank them politely for their concern and advice—and do what you want to do, guiltlessly.

Pitfall: "Every now and then I think: What the hell! My eating habits are getting sloppy."
Solution: Motivation slipping? Refer to the relevant chapters in this book, highlighting the sections that particularly pertain to you. Having the principles reinforced constantly will help you renew your commitment to stay thin.

Perhaps you need outside assistance. Enlist a friend to be your diet buddy, and call her whenever you're overwhelmed by the urge to overeat. Join a respected diet group, such as Weight Watchers or Overeaters Anonymous (OA), if you feel you'll benefit from the group support and if you're prepared to live and eat the way they instruct you to. (For example, Weight Watchers urges members to weigh and measure all their food strictly; OA insists that you commit your day's food plan to a "sponsor" whom you must telephone each day.) However, don't assume that just by paying your membership fees and attending meetings that your "work" will be simpler. It really won't be, but the support and understanding during this time may be exactly what you need.

Pitfall: "I've got a wedding (or vacation, or office party) coming up. How will I survive?"
Solution: These events—along with birthdays, anniversaries, baseball games, promotions, and the like—are all part of *life* and are meant to be enjoyed accordingly. *Not* to indulge yourself a bit on such occasions is self-deprivation of the highest order, especially when you're at or near your goal weight. You can enjoy them *if* you've done a little advance planning. Prepare to have that slice of cake or glass of champagne; just don't go hog-wild. Plan your days before the big event. Eat sensibly ahead of time, and step up your exercise after you've had the extra calories. Chances are you will have done your diet no real harm.

Pitfall: "At about three or four o'clock I get so hungry. Or maybe it's just that I'm bored and food is the first thing I go for."
Solution: Beware of boredom; it can be fat-producing. You can always snack on a no- or very-low-calorie food item, such as a diet soda or mineral water, or a carrot. A diverting activity will usually take your mind off eating until mealtime, so have such an activity ready at all times. You'll need an Alternative Activity List, containing a dozen or more things you enjoy doing that are

easy to jump right into the minute boredom rears its head. On that list might be:

- Continue (or start) working on a hobby or craft.
- Go to a neighborhood movie.
- Get your nails done.
- Check out your local library or bookstore.
- Call a friend.
- Watch TV (if the commercials don't tempt you to eat).

Being caught off-guard, with nothing to do *immediately,* can be dangerous. An Alternative Activity List will remind you of the fun things you like to do *besides* snacking and will head off those hunger pangs at the pass.

Pitfall: "Sometimes I feel so *deprived.* . . ."
Solution: Are you feeling deprived of *food,* or is it really something else you crave? You need to reward yourself period- ically during your maintenance phase, as you did during your weight-loss stage. Just because you're not *losing* weight doesn't mean you shouldn't reward yourself for *maintaining* it, via proper eating, exercise, and the like. Without a reward system you may not be sufficiently motivated to keep your weight stable at its current level, so devise for yourself an appropriate achievemen- t/reward plan, based on the suggestions on page 99.

More Tips for Staying on Track

- Be aware whenever you find yourself *stuffing your feelings* with food. If you're feeling mad, bad, or sad, just let yourself feel whatever the emotion is and trust yourself to get through it.

Writing down your thoughts and emotions, instead of burying them under a heavy "snack," is a good idea. The more you do this, the better you'll handle awful moods or moments in the future. Learn to *feel the feeling without the food*.

• Never feel obligated to eat any food you're offered simply to avoid hurting someone's feelings. If you *want* to eat it, fine; otherwise, politely say, "No, thanks" without explaining or apologizing for your diet.

• Put one favorite food on your "can't eat" list for one month. At the end of that time you'll either decide you can live without that food (and the extra calories), or you'll learn to have it in moderation.

• Tune out the negative comments. With this *same body* I've been told by "friends" that I should lose weight and by others that I look wonderful. Whom should I believe? I choose to believe only the praisers . . . and myself.

• Don't be so hard on yourself. Stop periodically to review and appreciate your dieting (and other!) accomplishments. The more you can acknowledge your day-to-day successes, the more likely you'll maintain your weight.

• After you reach your goal weight, choose a Red Flag Number, one not more than two to five pounds over your desired weight. The minute you spot that Red Flag Number on the scale, decide, right then and there, that you *must* turn things around by eating less and exercising more.

• If you typically devour every diet article you see in magazines and every new diet product you learn about on TV, stop and put yourself on a diet from diets for one month. See if you can get along without even paying attention to the newest fad diet. Try living with yourself, in your own body, and see how it feels. You may be pleasantly surprised at how much calmer and accepting of your body you are.

• Do the one diet thing you think you "can't" do. For me, I'd never been able to eat alone without reading or watching TV. But learning *just to eat* my meals—focusing on the food, without any distractions—has made me enjoy the food itself more and eat less because I can pay greater attention to when I'm really full.

• Eat before you go food shopping. Bring a shopping list and use it.

• If cooking makes you want to "sample" what you're preparing, keep a glass of water for sipping and a bowl of crudités for nibbling while you cook.

• Never apologize, never explain. No one has to know—and most people don't care—if you are or aren't on a diet. Your eating habits and body size are your business. Enough of "Oh, I *know* I shouldn't, but just this once . . ." or, "I've got to lose two more pounds. . . ." Even among diehard dieters, weight loss is a dull subject.

The Last 10 Pounds 10 Commandments

1. Thou shalt take responsibility for thy weight and eating habits.
2. Thou shalt take pleasure in the foods thou chooses to eat.
3. Thou shalt not apologize for thy eating behavior.
4. Honor thy healthy eating and regular exercise.
5. Thou shalt not kill a quart of ice cream.
6. Thou shalt give thyself a break from the torment of constant dieting.
7. Thou shalt not steal food off thy mate's plate.
8. Thou shalt remember that food has no power except that which thou gives it.
9. Thou shalt not covet thy neighbor's wife's figure.
10. Thou shalt love thyself always, regardless of thy weight.

VII

SPECIAL SITUATIONS

The Ex-Smoker's Last 10 Pounds

Are you an ex-smoker? Then you might be looking in the mirror these days thinking that your figure, which once resembled a slender, filter-tipped cigarette, now looks more like a short, stubby cigar.

The Atlanta, Georgia-based Centers for Disease Control (CDC) confirm a fear most smokers have: If they kicked the habit, they'd probably gain weight. In the CDC's study of 750 smokers who'd quit for a year or more, women averaged an eight-pound weight gain, with men putting on six pounds. The CDC also found that the amount of weight gained was in proportion to the number of cigarettes formerly smoked—the more smoked, the more weight added.

There's a physiological reason why the pounds may have started to creep up, even if you insist you haven't been eating more since you gave your butts the boot. According to David Krogh, author of *Smoking: The Artificial Passion,* nicotine increases metabolic rate, particularly when you're already engaged in some physical activity, so *lots* of calories are burned. Then you quit smoking, and what do you find? Your metabolism, so frisky under the influence of cigarettes, has now slowed down, and if you *do* start to nibble when you would otherwise be lighting up, it's a double whammy for your weight.

Furthermore, the quit smoking/gain weight issue tends to be more of a problem for women than for men. According to the U.S. surgeon general's 1988 report, women are more worried about weight gain after they give up smoking than men are. Perhaps that worry leads to overeating, because another survey David Krogh cites in his book indicates that female ex-smokers generally eat more than male ex-smokers.

Postsmoking weight gain isn't fun, and it's easy to get frustrated and unhappy about your extra pounds, but the situation's far from hopeless. You can drop the extra weight via one of the Last Ten Pounds Diets. And instead of reaching for a Milky Way when you'd normally reach for a Marlboro, chew sugarless or nicotine gum. (Be careful, though: Some people have found nicotine gum addictive.) "Smoke" on a plastic cigarette. Increase your water intake and munch on raw veggies, both of which will aid in digestion and elimination and help relieve that bloated feeling ex-smokers often get. Keep your idle hands busy with some sort of craft or hobby—even finger your rosary beads.

This may all sound like too much trouble, and one day it might seem a lot simpler just to resume smoking as a "diet aid." (Madison Avenue would love to have you believe that smoking equals slimness—have you *ever* seen an overweight woman in a cigarette ad?) However, I urge you to reconsider that plan. If your weight gain has been minimal and you don't choose to diet, then learn to live with it. Neil Grunberg, a professor of medical psychology at Uniformed Services University in Bethesda, Maryland, makes the point clearly: "If you quit smoking, you'll gain weight. But the serious health consequences of smoking far exceed the small danger from the 10 or so pounds you'll gain if you quit."

The New Mom's Last 10 Pounds

"With every baby I have, I gain 10 pounds!"

Sound familiar? It should. Many women who've never had a weight problem in their life suddenly find that the pounds have crept on—and stayed on—during pregnancy and after giving birth. And that's usually true whether or not you were one of those women who used your pregnancy as an excuse to party hearty. Now you discover, to your dismay, that your little seven- or eight-pound bundle of joy checked out of your womb leaving behind 10 or 15 pounds for *you* to deal with.

Women who are horrified to find themselves heavier after they give birth—particularly those who've always prided themselves on their good figures—tend to want to lose weight *now*. However, this is definitely not the time for any kind of strenuous dieting. Caring for your new baby puts stress on your body, and stringent dieting can lead to fatigue, poor health, and depression. Happily, though, your weight can come off in a reasonable length of time via a combination of sensible eating and simply letting nature take its course.

Marion McCartney, a certified nurse-midwife at Maternity Center Associates in Bethesda, Maryland, and coauthor of *The Midwife's Pregnancy and Childbirth Book,* points out that your postdelivery weight can be highly misleading. "Never get on a scale right after delivery—your weight can drop 12 pounds in 48 hours!" she warns. Give your body some time before you even *think* about dieting. "If brand-new mothers just waited two weeks," McCartney adds, "they'd automatically lose about 20 pounds," weight that is a combination of amniotic fluid, water from swelling, and extra blood. Assuming you gained the typical

25 to 30 pounds during your pregnancy, you'll then be left with about five to 10 pounds to lose (or more if you were already above your ideal weight at the time you became pregnant).

BREAST-FEEDING

There are lots of good reasons for breast-feeding your newborn; quicker weight loss is merely one of them. Not only does breast-feeding help you drop pounds fast, it also restores the uterus to its original size and gets your body back into shape. The 10-or-so-pound "fat pad" that magically appeared on your abdomen, back, and upper thighs during the second and third trimester of your pregnancy was designed solely as an energy store during breast-feeding. As a result, if you do breast-feed your baby and you're not overeating now, those extra 10 pounds may pretty much disappear within a couple of months—and without dieting.

Naturally, you'll want to follow your doctor's advice about what and how much to eat, especially if you're breast-feeding. She may tell you to increase your daily intake by as much as 1,000 calories for making breast milk, and she might also recommend iron and/or vitamin supplements. Even with the extra calories, you can probably still regain your girlish figure in a few months while eating well for two.

Marion McCartney recommends that, beginning about Week Three after delivery, you step on the scale once a week to see how your weight loss is progressing. Don't be surprised if things seem excruciatingly slow; that's normal. Says McCartney, "With the last 10 pounds, the weight often comes off in *ounces*." If you're one of the lucky moms shedding a safe one to two pounds a week, you're doing fine; if not, adjust your intake upward or downward accordingly. Above all, use common sense. As she points out, "Weight loss is such an individual thing. Some people drop it off all at once, while other women have a hard time losing weight. So much of it has to do with your own metabolism."

NON-BREAST-FEEDING MOMS

What if you're *not* breast-feeding, or simply want to be sure you're eating properly? The Last Ten Pounds Quick Diet, which allows for approximately 1,500 to 1,600 calories per day and a variety of nutritious foods, is a fine basic diet to follow. Just be certain to get your doctor's okay in case he has any special recommendations for you.

POSTPARTUM DEPRESSION AND OVEREATING

After the birth of your child, you'll certainly be exhausted, and you may experience postpartum depression. If you're the type of woman who usually turns to food in times of sadness or stress, be careful: Don't use your blue mood or fatigue as an excuse to overeat. Particularly now you'll find it easy to justify your overindulging. "What the hell," you're apt to say. "I'm already overweight/ It will take me forever to lose this weight/ I've been a blimp for the last nine months; what's another month of being fat?," etc. You get the picture.

Now's the time to find help for your depression. Talk to your doctor or midwife, or join a new-moms' support group. There you can openly discuss your feelings about motherhood, your new baby, your sex drive (or lack of it), and your body.

NEW-MOM EXERCISE

You'll be naturally more active after the baby arrives, so you'll be burning up many more calories than you did during the past nine months. But even if you've lost some weight just by playing mom, you've probably discovered to your dismay that you still can't slip into your jeans. That's because, regardless of what the scale says, your body has been stretched out and it's simply not the shape it once was. You know what that means: exercise.

Marian McCartney says you can begin doing some basic exercises at home to tighten your abdominal muscles as early as the day after a vaginal delivery. (Check with your doctor if you've had a cesarean; you'll need to be much more careful.) Start with stomach crunches: Lie on the floor with the small of your back flat on the floor, while slowly bringing your chin to your chest. Do these at the rate of one the first day, two the second day, etc. Keep things at a very moderate rate. If you find your exercising increases your bleeding, slow down, warns McCartney. Above all, keep asking yourself: "How am I feeling?" The answer to that question will help you pace yourself properly.

After a couple of weeks, you can start taking walks around the neighborhood or mall. After about six weeks, consider enrolling in an exercise class for new moms (with or without the baby). You'll find such classes given at local YWCAs and other locations; check the yellow pages under "Exercise." These classes aren't overly strenuous and will help ease you back into shape. Remember, it took you nine months to get your body ready to deliver your new baby, so don't get discouraged if it takes several months to return your body to its prepregnancy fitness level.

Your 10-Pounds-Overweight Mate

What, you may be asking, should you do about your slightly squishy spouse? Now that you've reached a resolution about *your* weight problem, what do you do about *his* or *hers*?

Nothing! If *you* want to lose weight, that's fine. But if your mate is sporting only a few extra pounds and doesn't seem particularly concerned about them, leave him alone! You've probably already tried nagging and coaxing him to diet and, as you've no doubt learned, it seldom works; a person will change only if *he* wants to or recognizes the benefits *himself*.

If you truly want to see him adjust his habits—and it's not wrong to be concerned that his weight situation might in time become more serious and affect his health and happiness—there *are* some steps you can take. Change your *own* eating habits and become a positive role model for him. Try *not* talking about this subject for a while. Instead, when it's your turn to do the cooking, quietly prepare meals for *both of you* that are healthy and lower in calories and fat. Eat sensibly in restaurants and on vacation. Ask your mate if he wants to join you when you go out for a walk or a bike ride, but don't force him or make him feel guilty if he doesn't.

Perhaps more than anything else, ask yourself why you regard your mate's few excess pounds as a problem in the first place. Is it really his *weight* you want him to change, or something else in his personality or behavior?

Take a good, hard look at your own motivation and goals before you make this into an opera. Have you convinced yourself that his body is a turn-off sexually? If his weight is only about 10 pounds more than it used to be, you should probably be exploring what's going on with *you* rather than forcing a diet on *him*. A wise woman once said, "If you really love the person, you love the body." If your affection for and attraction to your mate wavers as his stomach expands or contracts, then you must ask yourself that age-old Bee Gees question "How deep is your love?" Your mate has sustained his ardor for *you* while you've been 10 pounds overweight; can you not do the same for him?

Your 10-Pounds-Overweight Child

Take a look at yourself; then look at your child. If you (and/or your mate) are a bit overweight, chances are your youngster is, too. A coincidence? Probably not. As stated earlier, a child with an overweight parent has a 40 percent chance of being overweight himself, and one with two overweight parents doubles his own odds for obesity.

How does this happen? Children of overweight parents tend to be born with bigger or more fat cells, and the larger the number and size of these cells, the greater a person's chance of getting and staying fat. But it's not *all* heredity; environment plays a major role, too, for even *adopted* children tend to get chubby if their adoptive folks are that way themselves.

An overweight child is seldom a happy one. If *your* 10 pounds sometimes feel heavy on *you,* imagine what the extra weight must seem like on your son or daughter. And if you think about those negative feelings you've had in the past about your weight, you'll get a pretty good sense of how your child feels—even if he never says a word about it.

Many parents of chubby children blame themselves, but the guilt might not always be warranted. Perhaps it's *not* the size of the portions you serve at home or the availability of junk food in your cupboards. Maybe your child snacks too much during or after school, or is eating too much of certain foods and too little of others. Maybe he prefers video games to volleyball and doesn't exercise enough to burn off calories. In any case, you *do* need to question why your child seems to get most of his pleasure from eating—and your role in his pattern.

Now's the time to get to the heart of the matter, without causing your child further shame or embarrassment about his weight. You might be unconsciously contributing to his poor eating habits, and just as *you're* trying to lick your own 10-pound problem, you want to help him do so, too, in a loving and caring way—and get him on the right track to a lifetime of sound eating habits.

Don't expect it to be easy, though. According to Dr. Daniela Alloro, Ph.D., of Contemporary Psychology Associates, a Los Angeles-based psychologist who works with children and adolescents in treatment for eating disorders, "diet" is a dirty word for most kids. "It's difficult enough for an adult to feel deprived; for a child, it's much worse. Children aren't good at delaying gratification and making a sacrifice *now* for a reward later on," she explains. "There's also the matter of peer pressure for a child of about nine or 10. When he's older, especially when he's in his teens, it's difficult to go to a movie or a dance with friends and not eat something. When kids go out, it's generally to McDonald's or a similar place, and it can be embarrassing for the child to have to say, 'I can't eat. I'm on a diet.' "

Realizing the challenge that lies ahead for you and your child, you first must be absolutely certain that he even *needs* to lose weight. Says Dr. Alloro, "The younger the child, the more important it is to get your doctor's advice about a diet, because of the higher rate of growth in the early years. It's crucial that the child's muscles and bones, circulatory and other systems are nourished properly." In an older child, a too-low-calorie diet might cause a serious vitamin deficiency or even anemia. So get your doctor's okay on how much, if any, weight your child should lose and what combination of diet and increased activity will accomplish it. Once you get the go-ahead, these tips should help:

1. Avoid using the word "diet." Kids hate the ideas of do's, don'ts, and deprivation.

2. Let your child know you're in this *together*. Show him that, while you're adjusting his serving sizes and selections, you're doing the same for yourself.

3. Set a good example. Your child will be less likely to overeat if she sees you eating properly and you're at a sensible weight, too.

4. Don't just focus on your child's eating; encourage him to get more exercise as a way to step up his metabolic rate and lose pounds. "Increased activity should be viewed as a game, not a task," insists Dr. Alloro. Go out with him one or two afternoons a week for a bike ride, a neighborhood jog, or some one-on-one basketball in the schoolyard. On weekends, instead of the family's heading for the usual movie or restaurant, have a picnic, where physical activity can be part of the afternoon's events. You'll *all* benefit, physically and emotionally, from this time together.

5. Talk to your child and find out what, besides the meals you prepare at home, he's eating, and when. Perhaps you can adjust the at-home meal schedule so he will be less inclined to snack on junk food when he gets hungry.

6. Ask her what she *really* likes to eat, and occasionally incorporate some of her favorites, such as pizza, into your regular meals.

7. Instead of saying, "You can't eat this!"—which will only make your child want it more—use food substitutions. For instance, instead of ice cream, serve frozen yogurt, which has a similar taste and texture but fewer calories and less fat. Avoid dramatic (and upsetting) statements such as, "No more ice cream for you!"

8. Let her come up with a menu plan for one meal each week, so she can feel greater control over her own eating habits and have more of the foods she enjoys.

9. Don't criticize how or what he's eating. Instead of "Jason, that's your *third* helping of potatoes!" say, "Jason, why don't you have some more salad if you're still hungry?"

10. Don't insist she clean her plate. Even if you *have* spent hours preparing a special dish, you'll all be better off if you wrap up and store the leftovers than force your child to down every last morsel.

11. Dinner-table stress is a major cause of overeating. Make sure mealtime is pleasant for the whole family and not loaded with highly emotional conversation or bickering.

12. Strive as much as possible for a regular, fixed dinner hour each night, with all family members seated at the table. Your child will learn better eating habits this way than if the "dinner hour" is different for each person, with one in front of the TV, one nibbling at the kitchen counter, etc.

13. Investigate your child's school lunch and snack program. For example, some public schools have switched to lower-calorie/lower-fat items, such as low-fat milk. If your child has a

choice, teach him how and why to make smart food selections at school. And if you're not happy with what's provided at school, prepare healthy brown-bag lunches for him.

14. Break the habit of rewarding or soothing your child with food. It will only teach her to "handle" her emotions by eating, a habit you're probably now trying to break yourself.

15. Is his overeating due to some stress or change at school or with friends? Let him know you're there to discuss any problems or concerns he has, and show him how to deal with anxiety without food.

16. If your teenage daughter is dieting, make sure she really needs to lose weight. Peer pressure and the desire to be superslim—rather than a true weight problem—may be causing her to reduce her intake drastically. If she's already at a normal weight and she wants to drop four or five pounds, instead of getting into an argument, say, "Okay, what can I do to help you with your meals?" But if she tries to lose substantially more weight, this may indicate the onset of anorexia—and that's pathological. "There's no way the family can handle it alone," says Dr. Alloro.

17. Stop communicating your own food obsessions to your child. Certainly it would be lovely if your son just *naturally* preferred cauliflower to Kit Kat bars, but even if he doesn't, you can calmly and nonjudgmentally guide him to making better food selections.

18. Don't punish your child (as you may be punishing yourself) with the we'll-do-it-after-you-lose-weight mentality. Take your daughter out *this week* for a pretty new outfit; don't say, "Let's

wait till you get a little thinner." Life is happening *right now;* it shouldn't be put on hold until your child is the "perfect" weight.

A Word About Anorexia and Bulimia

Being 10 pounds overweight isn't cause for too much alarm for most of us. Yet from time to time, a simple 10-pound weight problem can get severely out of hand and develop into one of the life-threatening conditions known as anorexia nervosa or bulimia.

Anorexia is a self-starvation, and bulimia is the pattern of gorging and purging (forced vomiting or the excessive use of laxatives or diuretics) as a form of weight loss or maintenance. Both anorexics and bulimics tend to be women with highly distorted body images who view themselves as fat, regardless of their actual size. Both groups are terrified that anything they eat—even if it's just a peanut or a radish—will make them grossly overweight. Anorexics are frequently "model children," growing up with a drive for perfectionism and overachievement.

In terms of eating patterns, anorexics may diet so strenuously that they eventually stop eating almost completely. Consequently, they may lose as much as 25 percent of their body weight over a short period of time. Bulimics usually remain closer to an acceptable body weight. (An article on eating disorders in the May 13, 1991, issue of *Newsweek* states that most bulimics are within 10 pounds of their normal body weight.) Bulimics may begin their habit of purging merely as a way of avoiding the calories from a particularly large meal, but soon it develops into an excuse to binge. "Hey, I can eat all I want and not get fat!" is the typical thinking, and as long as there's no fear that the weight will stay on, the pattern continues—sometimes with harmful results.

According to Dr. Daniela Alloro, who works with anorexic and bulimic clients in her Los Angeles practice, "Some of my patients start off saying, 'I'm a little chubby.' So they diet to try to lose five to six pounds. But then losing weight becomes an obsession, and they continue to diet until they become anorexic." She says that the origins of this pattern aren't yet clear, but one thing is certain: It's a habit that can wreak havoc with your health and, in the most extreme cases, can cause death.

If you're currently engaging in this dangerous game of weight-loss Russian roulette, or believe this is your only route to a slimmer body, you need more help than this book can provide. Consult a mental-health professional as soon as possible.

VIII

MAYBE YOU'RE
NOT REALLY OVERWEIGHT

Look at these statistics:

• An article on eating disorders in the May 13, 1991, issue of *Newsweek* stated that nearly one-fifth of women between ages 18 and 29 are trying to lose weight *even though they don't need to.*

• In a 1986 Harris Poll survey, 96 percent of the respondents said *they wanted to change something about their body.* Among the women surveyed, 78 percent said they *would like to change their weight.*

• In a 1984 *Glamour* magazine reader survey, 42 percent of the 33,000 respondents said they would *rather lose 10 or 15 pounds than find success in romance or a career.*

How do you know if you're 10 pounds overweight, anyway? Certainly you have indicators of your own, but . . . just listen. It seems as though everyone and everything are telling you, in so many words, that you need to go on a diet:

• *Family members*. *They* know what's best for you. You'd look and feel better a few pounds lighter, they insist. The kids joke about your "healthy" appetite.

• *"Friends."* You've started hearing things such as, "Hey, buddy, looks like marriage agrees with you!" accompanied by a "good-natured" poke in the stomach or, "It's hard to watch what you eat when you're home with a new baby, isn't it?"

• *Coworkers*. People at the office who are *thinner* than you are swigging Ultra Slim-Fast and slipping out at 4:45 P.M. for their sessions at Jack LaLanne. (And weren't they staring at you just a *little* as you polished off that meatball hero for lunch?)

• *The doc*. Cholesterol's up, and the gut's a bit bigger than it was the last time you were there. But *wait* a minute: Isn't your doctor *heavier* than you are?

• *Clothes*. That damn clothes dryer! You fit into most of your "regular" outfits these days—but some you don't.

• *Standardized charts*. Some people swear by 'em, and if their weight doesn't fall within the range set for their height and gender, they announce, "Time to diet!"

• *Everyday things*. What was once accomplished with ease— say, climbing a couple of flights of stairs—now leaves you breathless and ready for the BarcaLounger and the remote-control channel changer.

• *"They."* "They" say you should be thin for the wedding or the reunion or any other landmark event that involves lots of photo opportunities. "They" also say you can't get a man unless you're superslim.

• *Hollywood/the media*. Weight-loss guru Dr. Kelly D. Brownell estimates that most actresses and models probably have a body-fat composition of 10 to 15 percent, comparable to that of distance runners. Normal body fat for healthy women is about twice that: 22 to 26 percent.

• *Society*. The 1991 movie *Eating* convincingly made the case that it's hard to be a women today and cope with society's incessant demands on their appearance, creating standards for physical perfection that rarely apply to men. As the movie's director, Harry Jaglom, says:

> Men aren't given the daily message that their success in finding love and fulfillment revolves around the number of inches they can take off their waist or hips. No man is told by society that his essential worth is nonexistent because he doesn't look "right" in a bathing suit. Quite simply, men don't have it hammered into them from their earliest childhood that happiness and all the good things in life can only be bought by starving themselves. Food and eating, I have come to see, are a metaphor for how incredibly difficult and painful and complicated it is to be a woman in our society. How truly *hard* it is for women to survive reasonably intact. And how triumphant that seemingly simple act of survival really is.

Society's pressures on a woman to conform to a level of thinness that not only may be unrealistic for her but also *changes* periodically and arbitrarily has been addressed in two excellent books. They are the classic *Fat Is a Feminist Issue* by Susie Orbach and the more recent *The Beauty Myth* by Naomi Wolf. Both are worth a read.

Who says you need to lose weight? A lot of people, apparently. But if it's not *you* who's saying it, then maybe the "advice" is better ignored.

Ten Reasonable Reasons
to Keep Those Last 10 Pounds

1. Most current medical findings indicate that being 10 pounds above normal body weight is not considered a health risk.
2. You look fine . . . or better.
3. You're eating fairly healthfully and exercise at least a couple of times a week.
4. Your doctor hasn't uncovered any substantial medical problems.
5. Your clothes fit you decently.
6. The extra weight really doesn't stop you from doing anything you want to do.
7. You feel comfortable at this weight.
8. Trying to sustain a lower weight in the past has been very difficult or impossible for you.
9. You enjoy eating.
10. In the scope of all the problems in your life, this is not one of your biggest.

As a further way to help you decide whether or not to remain at your present weight, ask yourself these questions:

• *How do I think my life-style will change or improve once I reach my desired weight? Are my expectations realistic?* You may be wondering: *What if my life doesn't get dramatically better when I'm thinner?* Hint: It probably won't. Be ready for the usual disappointments, setbacks, and obstacles you had before. However (and this is a big however), you may find you're now able to handle them with greater ease and confidence.

• *Is there anything I can do right now, at my present weight, to help achieve some of my goals?* Losing 10 pounds may be *one* task you've set for yourself. What are the others? Are there any small steps you can take *today,* before you reach your desired weight, to change your life for the better?

If it's a new job you want, call friends to see if there are any openings they've heard about, or update your résumé and get new ones printed by the end of next week.

Want a relationship? Ask your buddies to throw an informal party where you can be exposed to some new faces, take an adult-ed course, or join a club. Remember, you don't *have* to be the "perfect weight" to start taking charge of your life.

• *What am I prepared to do or give up to maintain my new, lower weight?* Something has to give! Are you *really* ready to live with different eating and exercising patterns? Prepared to make food sacrifices and time (for exercise) sacrifices? You *must* if you intend to be successful in the long term.

• *Am I ready to stop kidding myself about what I will or won't be able to do as a thinner person?* Do you think being thin means you can overeat without eventually paying the price? *Hey! I wear a size 10 now! I can eat this ice cream sundae!* (Yes, but not every day.)

Or do you have irrational fears about living—and eating—in the real world? *I can never eat out again!* or, *I can't possibly go to that wedding/party/shower. Who knows what they'll serve?* (If losing the last 10 pounds means you can never feel comfortable around food, then you must ask yourself: Is it really worth it?)

MAYBE YOU SHOULDN'T LOSE THOSE LAST 10 POUNDS

That's the question you'll ultimately have to answer for yourself. But talking strictly from a health standpoint, experts have very definite opinions.

"Losing the last 10 pounds is not important to health; it's just cosmetic," Dr. Xavier Pi-Sunyer of Columbia University believes. "I'm not enthusiastic about people losing it. First, there's little data to suggest that being 10 pounds overweight causes an excess risk; only if people are obese (more than 20 to 25 percent above their normal weight) does the health risk kick in. Second, not everyone is biologically programmed the same way, which is why the height/weight tables have a wide range of acceptability. I may be 5' 8" and weigh 160, while someone else of the same height may weigh 150, and we may both be at the right weight given the differences in our body composition, frame, size, genetic composition, fat distribution, and so on. Slavishly trying to come up with an ideal weight for everyone is silly. Many individuals, particularly women, focus on a goal weight that's idealized and which, in their present situation and in society, may be considered normal but may actually be for them abnormal, that is, underweight. For a lot of people, the last 10 pounds are really the first 10 pounds of underweight."

Thomas Wadden, Ph.D., associate professor of psychology at the University of Pennsylvania School of Medicine, goes on to remind people that there are really only two smart reasons to lose weight: (1) to reduce health complications and (2) to achieve a weight that makes sense given your particular history of weight loss and gain. Think about what's a *reasonable weight* for you to achieve, he says, then take the appropriate action. His rule of thumb for determining a proper body weight: Aim for the lowest weight that you've maintained for a year or more since age 21 *without excessive dieting,* even if that number is 10 or 20 pounds over your weight at 21.

Dr. Pi-Sunyer adds that this "settling weight" will be the one at which your body feels most comfortable. Even if it's about 10 pounds over your desired weight "it's probably acceptable—at least there's no evidence that it's bad for you," he notes.

The experts conclude that if you want to lose 10 pounds but are not sure you can *keep* them off, perhaps it's just not wise to lose the weight in the first place.

A Little More to Love

People determined to diet off those last 10 pounds will find in these pages three detailed diet plans, exercise information, words of encouragement, savvy suggestions from successful dieters, strategies for weight maintenance: the works.

But what if you've decided that you *don't* want to diet any longer, that you'll keep those last 10 pounds, to have and to hold, from this day forth? Well, *you'll* need some support and encouragement, too—maybe even more than the dieters. Why? Because it takes grit and self-confidence to say, firmly and deliberately, "I'm fine just the way I am. I may not be model-thin, but I don't *need* that to be happy."

If such is your choice, it is indeed a brave one, because it flies in the face of much of what's going on in your world today. Your newfound attitude and determination notwithstanding, you're *still* going to be surrounded by chronic calorie-counters, frenetic label-readers, and all-weather joggers. You're going to find yourself in the company of women who compliment one another on how skinny they have become, and when they get around to noticing you, they'll quickly change the subject. You'll continue to get an occasional "playful" poke in the gut, and there'll always be that moment (or evening) of insecurity about your body as you disrobe for a new lover. Face it: Maintaining your present weight level means you'll never be the slimmest one on the beach, at the cocktail party, or in the locker room.

Can you live with that? Because if you *can't,* you'll drive yourself crazy—and probably to a binge or two that will send your weight soaring beyond the 10-pound mark. But if you *can* accept yourself (and your weight) as you are—and it seems as though you have—you can discover a new serenity, a sudden peacefulness within you that you never knew existed. Finally, you'll be able to get on with your life and focus on what really matters to you. Without obsessing about your few extra pounds, you may actually find you have more time than you know what to do with, regardless of your present schedule and responsibilities.

In short, you'll have a big weight off of you.

If you *do* go this route, I'm not saying to abandon all reason, eat heedlessly, and disregard the bathroom scale altogether. Eat what you want, but use good, common sense. Exercise regularly, even if it's just a 20-minute walk after dinner or a brisk morning run around the park with the dog. Hop on the scale once a month or so, just to be certain you haven't *exceeded* those 10 pounds. Periodically review this book for a quick refresher course in the basics, and when you feel your eating/exercise habits are starting to get sloppy, follow the Last Ten Pounds Quick Diet to get yourself back on track.

And if you do decide to live with the weight, congratulate yourself—for giving yourself a break, and for having the smarts and the courage to follow your head instead of the herd.

Ten Reasons to be Glad
You're (Only) 10 Pounds Overweight

Okay, so you're starting to get used to the idea that staying a bit over your "ideal" weight isn't such a bad idea. Let's take a moment here to appreciate the fact that your current situation is actually a pretty enviable one. *Lots* of people wish they had only 10 pounds to lose. Particularly if you've just concluded a long dieting period and you've already shed a good deal of weight, it's *crucial* that you take the time to give yourself a mental pat on the back for a job well done.

So right now you can enjoy the fact that:

1. You probably look fine right now.
2. You can probably fit into most of the clothes you like.
3. You're most likely not endangering your health (or else your health has already improved from the weight you've lost so far).
4. People think you look pretty good (or you've already begun receiving compliments for the weight you've dropped).
5. You're active (or at least don't have a lot of excess weight as an excuse *not* to be).
6. You can find your size in most "ordinary" clothing and department stores.
7. Catching your reflection in a shop window or in your bedroom mirror isn't cause for too much alarm, or is even a pleasant experience.
8. People on the street aren't staring at you (and if you *think* they are, it's either your imagination or your toupé is askew).

9. You don't need to ask for an "extender" for your airplane seat belt.

10. Waiters don't bat an eyelash when you order dessert.

Looking Better Without Dieting: (Almost) Painless Firming Exercises

You're sticking with your last 10 pounds, and you don't want to engage in any heavy-duty workouts. Fine. But you *can* improve your health, your appearance, and your state of mind without dieting if you get in some brisk walking as often as possible. And for a simple little way to help you look slimmer *right now,* try *standing straight.*

Mom was right: Posture really *can* make a difference in how you look, and that's especially true if you're just a few pounds over your "ideal" weight. You can actually *disguise* those extra pounds if your posture is good and you stand, walk, and sit with your head tall and your back straight. You'll also appear more self-confident—not a bad thing no matter what you weigh.

In addition, you can begin doing *firming* exercises to help tone your body and enhance its overall appearance. (Remember, these will not *burn calories,* as aerobic exercises will.) A dozen simple exercises, created by fitness therapist Cal Pozo, are described below. Do them while holding two- to three-pound weights in each hand. (Buy dumbbells at a sporting goods store, or use detergent or bleach containers emptied of their original contents and filled with water or sand until they weigh two to three pounds, or whatever you are comfortable with.) Run through the series three times a week for best results.

1. *For upper arms.* Stand with feet slightly apart, upper arms close to the sides of your body, and fists clenched and held

straight forward, as if you were holding on to ski poles. Keeping upper arms close to your sides, move your fists as far behind you as possible. Return to original position. Do 10 to 20 times.

2. *For arms, shoulders, upper back, and waist.* Stand with feet apart, toes pointing outward, elbows bent and pointing downward, dumbbells held at shoulder level. Reach up high with the left dumbbell, straightening your arm while twisting your trunk to the right. As you start to lower the dumbbell back to the original position, twist your trunk to the left while reaching up high with the right dumbbell. Do 10 to 15 times per side.

3. *For upper torso and waist.* Stand with feet apart, arms held straight out at shoulder level, perpendicular to your torso. Keeping your lower body fixed and arms straight, twist your upper body to the left, as far over as possible, then back to the original position, then twist to the right as far as possible. Do 10 to 20 times.

4. *For upper and lower back.* Stand with feet apart, toes pointing outward, and arms straight down in front of your trunk, both hands grasping the globes of one of the dumbbells. Turn your shoulders to the left and bend down, touching your left foot with the dumbbell, rounding your spine slowly, and gradually straightening your spine as you return to an upright position. Repeat, turning shoulders and bending down to the right. Exhale on your way down, inhale while coming back up. Do 10 to 15 times per side.

5. *For back, arms, shoulders, and legs.* Stand with feet slightly apart, holding each dumbbell in one hand on either side of your trunk, back flat (not hunched), and face forward. Squat slightly, bending your knees and raising the dumbbells out to shoulder level. Lowering the dumbbells, slowly return to the original position.

Inhale on your way up, exhale on your way down. Do 10 to 20 times.

6. *For stomach and lower back.* Stand with feet together and hands on hips (or one hand holding the back of a chair for support). Alternate raising knees high up to the chest. Do 10 to 20 times per leg.

7. *For bust, stomach, and thighs.* Lie on your back, with legs straight and together on the floor, arms stretched overhead on the floor, a dumbbell in each hand. Bring both knees to your chest while raising the dumbbells until your arms are perpendicular to your trunk at the shoulders. Lower your arms and legs to your original position. Exhale as you raise your knees, inhale as you lower them. Do 10 to 20 times.

8. *For upper arms and thighs.* Stand with feet and arms as in Exercise 1. Squat slightly as you raise your elbows to shoulder level. Return to the original position. Do 15 to 20 times.

9. *For hips and outer thighs.* Stand next to a chair, grasping the top for balance. Keep your legs slightly apart, with your weight on the leg closer to the chair. Keeping your outer leg straight, raise it out to the side, as high as it can go. Then return to the original position. Do 20 times per leg.

10. *For hips and inner and outer thighs.* Stand next to a chair, as in Exercise 9. Keeping your outer leg straight, swing it back and forth in front of the inner leg, as if you were swinging a golf club, as far in either direction as it can go. Do 20 full swings per leg.

11. *For thighs.* Stand with heels together and raised, toes pointing out, a dumbbell in each hand at each hip. Keeping your

trunk vertical, bend your knees, pointing out, until you're half-squatting. Stop when your heels start to lift up off the floor. Then slowly raise yourself up to your original position. Exhale while going down, inhale while coming back up. Do 10 to 20 times.

12. *For calves and thighs.* Stand with feet together and arms at sides. Lift yourself up on your toes, raising your arms up at either side to shoulder level. Then return to the starting position. Do 25 to 30 times.

Maintenance if You're Remaining at Your Present Weight

1. Continue your current eating pattern, emphasizing a balanced, nutritious diet.
2. Exercise aerobically 30 minutes per day, as many days a week as possible.
3. Record foods and feelings in the Last Ten Pounds Success Diary as often as desired.
4. Weigh in at least once a month.
5. Plan on maintaining this weight forever.

Eight More Ways
to Live Happily with Your Last 10 Pounds

1. *Go to a spa.* If you can afford it (and they're *not* all superexpensive), there's nothing more pleasurable. True, you'll be put on a strict food regime and be expected to work up a daily sweat, but the wonderfully pampering pedicures, massages, and

herbal wraps will more than make up for any feeling of deprivation. (You'll also see people a lot heavier than you are.)

2. *Put romantic (read dim) lighting near your mirror.* You'll be amazed at how thin you look.

3. *Find a mate who loves you just the way you are.* If you don't already have one, there are plenty of potential mates around. Keep looking and don't get discouraged.

4. *Get busy.* Take up a hobby—reading, needlepoint, sex, canoeing, painting-by-numbers—that you truly enjoy and that lets you forget about eating. Once you get into the flow of your favorite activity, overeating will lose its importance in your life.

5. *Have an affair (or end the one you're having).* Both are time-honored ways to lose one's appetite, and you can always fall in love again. (A bonus: You'll be a little slimmer the next time around.)

6. *Change your looks.* Do something fairly drastic—chop off or dye your hair if you're a woman, grow (or shave off) a beard or mustache if you're a man. You'll start hearing comments such as, "Say . . . What's *different* about you? Did you lose weight?" (And, of course, always answer "Yes!")

7. *Move into a larger house or apartment.* (You'll feel smaller.)

8. *Volunteer for a worthwhile cause.* Sign up to work a few hours a week manning a crisis hot line or helping out at a shelter for the homeless. Your 10 pounds will seem extraordinarily trivial by comparison, and you'll be glad you decided to ignore them for good.

Twenty-Five Successful People
Who Never Bothered to Lose Their Last 10 Pounds
(and Probably Haven't Lost Sleep Over It)

1. Bea Arthur
2. Jay Leno
3. The Queen Mother
4. Homer Simpson
5. Robin Leach
6. Frank Sinatra
7. Eleanor Roosevelt
8. Walter Matthau
9. Norman Mailer
10. Ethel Merman
11. Carroll O'Connor
12. Bette Midler
13. Telly Savalas
14. Mae West
15. General Colin Powell
16. Aretha Franklin
17. Ed Asner
18. Raisa Gorbachev
19. Beverly Sills
20. Shelley Winters
21. Barbara Bush
22. Julia Child
23. Andy Rooney
24. Erma Bombeck
25. James Earl Jones

The Slimming Powers of Self-Confidence

One evening last year, I attended a meeting of my writers' group in an elegant midtown restaurant. During the cocktail reception I found myself seated at a table opposite a fellow member I had known by name and reputation but had never formally met. Instantly I noticed how attractive she was, with a gorgeous mane of brown hair cascading over her body-hugging, intriguingly-colored seafoam-green dress.

We began chatting about editors and publishers, and during

that time I got a good opportunity really to examine her. I admired her appearance, right down to the multicolored sandals and pedicured toes I spotted out of the corner of my eye. What's more, I found her bright, perceptive, and funny, easily able to make me laugh a half-dozen times in the 15 or so minutes we were together. And despite the time and attention she had clearly devoted to putting herself together, never once during our conversation did she give in to an urge to smooth her hair or check her appearance in the mirror just behind me. In short, she displayed tremendous self-confidence, and I was extremely impressed, if not slightly envious.

Eventually she excused herself politely, and as she stood up to leave, it was impossible to ignore her derrière, which was not simply large—it was *enormous*. Okay, I thought, so she has a big butt. Yet if this woman felt the least bit embarrassed or apologetic about it, *I* couldn't tell, and I seriously doubted whether anyone else could either. Everything about her seemed to say, "I like who I am and I like the way I look, and if you're smart, you should, too!"

The point of relating this little anecdote is to illustrate a theory I've long held: *Self-confidence makes you thin*. In fact, self-confidence makes you anything you want to be: beautiful, smart, witty, kind, passionate . . . and the perfect weight for *you*. Self-confidence can fool the eye about the size of your hips better than any black dress or girdle can. If you possess self-confidence, you don't need a bathroom scale, or a shelf full of diet books, or a micrometer to measure the width of your protein bread. If you have self-confidence, you need never be on a diet again.

Those people who've spent a lifetime counting calories and doing push-ups would be far better off working on developing their personality, their relationships, their career objectives, their interests . . . and their self-confidence. If your own self-confidence is in place, it's easy to accept who you are—and what you weigh. And, like the woman described above, you probably radiate satisfaction with yourself—and challenge *anyone* to dare to say you need to lose 10 pounds.

IX

FINAL THOUGHTS

What would it feel like never again to worry about those last 10 pounds, to avoid for the rest of your life the agony of "What did I do? Did I really eat all *that*?" Wouldn't it be glorious, as if a tremendous weight (pun very much intended) had been lifted from you forever?

You *can* know that feeling, and enjoy it for the rest of your days. In fact, you could have had it even *before* you picked up this book. It's sort of like when the Good Witch told Dorothy in *The Wizard of Oz,* "You always had the power to go back to Kansas, but you wouldn't have believed me before—you had to learn it for yourself." If *The Last Ten Pounds* has given you that knowledge and helps you put it into practice in your day-to-day life, then it's done its job.

I hope that by now you've come truly to believe that *deliberately choosing* to remain a size 12, rather than continue the struggle to be a size 6, is perfectly acceptable and valid, and doesn't in any way detract from your value as a human being. You are a good person, whether you eat that extra handful of peanuts or not, and a 10-pounds-skinnier body will not, in all likelihood, dramatically affect your world. You'll still occasionally fight with your husband, you'll get that raise, you'll have a terrific vacation, your kids will drive you nuts: In short, life will go on, more or less as it always has. The main difference: You can now eat in peace. You can appreciate the fact that food is not only nourishment and fuel for your body but also *delicious* and one of the pleasures of being alive.

The way your body looks is and always has been your own decision. You can *allow* other people, or magazine photos, or TV commercials, or the scale to convince you that you need to lose weight—or you can choose to listen to your own head and heart and not make the 10 or so pounds the tragedy of your life. Admittedly it's hard to go against the tide of opinion that says Thin Is In. But if you're only 10 pounds over your "ideal" weight, you *are* sufficiently thin.

Hold your head up, stop apologizing for what you eat, and be proud of who you are—no matter what you weigh.

My Story

When I was a little girl, my mother's weight was a constant source of embarrassment to me. I cringed at the thought of being spotted with her, lumbering down the street in her Lane Bryant special, by one of my second-grade classmates. I carried around a single terrifying scenario in my head: Pretty 'n' blonde Janet Cook and cute 'n' freckled Karen Kramer would see me with my mother on our way to Key Food or the dentist's office. The girls would emit a nervous, "Hi," then rush off so they could giggle and whisper (but loud enough for me to hear), "Did you see *that*?"

Actually, I needn't have worried so much; there was scant chance this scene would ever get played out. Mom was loath to leave the house, partly out of self-consciousness, partly because it was hard for her to walk. As a result, there were remarkably few Saturday afternoon mother/daughter shopping trips as I was growing up. We were the only family I knew of living in the New York metropolitan area—the fashion capital of the world—who ordered their clothing from a Spiegel catalog. On those rare occasions when I found myself in a department store, it was usually accompanied by some other relative.

Mom wasn't just being lazy. Her weight created chronic health problems for her—ruptured hernias, mostly. My father, older brother, Calvin, and I were always at the ready in case of one of her frequent attacks, which invariably meant a middle-of-the-night trip to the hospital emergency room. There my pale, trembling mother would commonly be mistaken for my grandmother.

My mother weighs 315 pounds. It's a weight she's more or less sustained her entire adult life. But for all Mom's struggles with pantyhose, movie-theater seats, and subway turnstiles, I've long understood that her weight problem is *my* problem, too. I've never been more than about 20 pounds above my goal. But when you have a 315-pound parent, your "weight problem" is generally more in your head than on the bathroom scale.

When you have an overweight parent, eating and not eating become your daily obsessions. People like me study height/weight charts, know the calorie counts of everything from roast pig to Raisinettes, and can furnish detailed reports of the food-related deaths of Karen Carpenter and "Mama" Cass Elliott. We own as many diet books as cookbooks, a frayed tape measure, and a multiple-sized wardrobe "just in case" of a weight fluctuation. And God knows mine has fluctuated: from the 10 minutes when I weight 119 pounds following some serious dieting in the mid 1970s to the agonizing month during the summer of 1988 when I hovered around 145.

As I've discovered with some measure of pain, growing up with an overweight parent shapes not only your body but also your beliefs—about yourself, the world, and your place in it.

My mother always considered her cooking her biggest selling point as a wife and mother, not surprising for a woman of her generation. Food was a leitmotiv in our home: We had the standard-issue bowl of waxed fruit as a table centerpiece, and kitchen wallpaper featuring clusters of cherries. Decades into their marriage, Mom, glowing like a new bride, would talk about how much Daddy still loved her pot roasts and lemon meringue pies. Our family ate simply but well. "Your father works hard; he likes to eat meat when he comes home" was an oft-heard remark. Mom also shopped for many more than the four of us—she believed that hungry folks were always hovering, waiting to be fed, and it was vital to be prepared for the company that frequently dropped by.

Nevertheless, though we were constantly surrounded by food, my father, brother, and I somehow managed to remain at a normal weight. Daddy and Calvin were blessedly born with speedy metabolisms, and they readily burned off whatever they ate. As for me, I never had a particular desire to stuff myself as a kid, and Mom was sensitive enough not to be a food-pusher. I remember her telling me, "Watch out—I don't want you to look like me" more often than "Eat! Eat!"

But Mom's own ability to distance herself from food was sorely limited. For instance, she tended to snack whenever she got depressed or felt "weak." "Getting depressed" could be the result of a tiff with her sister Dorothy, who lived upstairs, or *TV Guide* arriving in the mail two days late. On Yom Kippur, the holiday when Jews traditionally fast for 24 hours, my mother would last for about 10 of them, at which time we'd start to hear the rustle of the white–bread bag and the hum of the electric can opener. Sure enough, Mom, "feeling faint," would be preparing herself an early lunch.

Sooner or later, she'd go on a diet. No weight-loss book, pill, powder, or machine escaped her notice. Our kitchen counter was gradually transformed into her personal pharmacy, covered with potions promising to melt away fat. When those didn't work, she moved on to low-calorie cookbooks, Weight Watchers classes, and tricks such as "hiding" the leftover roast chicken from herself by wrapping it in tinfoil and tucking it in the far reaches of the fridge. (But Mom was too smart; she always found that chicken!)

As successful as Mom was as a cook and homemaker, she was a dismal failure as a dieter. Daddy, Calvin, and I, her biggest cheerleaders at the start of each new weight-loss program, turned sarcastic or silent when the day inevitably came that she resumed her postdinner or late-night nibbling. Again and again, she'd concoct some feeble excuse for why this month's Miracle Diet failed her—a leak ruined her kitchen linoleum, or a friend bad-mouthed her behind her back, and she was simply too angry or upset to control her eating. Up to a point, we were sympathetic—we knew she had tried, and we were well aware how self-conscious her body made her feel. But the afternoon Calvin and I returned home from school and caught her "snacking" her way through a box of Ayds dietetic candies was the day we knew her case was hopeless. Month after month, year after year, Mom stayed fat.

I, meanwhile, remained slender as I left my teens and entered my twenties. But once I graduated from college, took a part-time office job, and launched my writing career, the extra pounds mysteriously started to creep up. My nice, 125-pound body was soon a distant memory as I inched my way to 130 and beyond. Now I had to shift my attention from my mother's weight problem to my own; it could no longer be ignored.

I began noticing that whenever I'd had a fight with my

boyfriend or was nervous about a job interview or agonized over getting an apartment, I'd overeat—just like Mom! Because I was constantly nagging my mother about *her* rotten eating habits, I had to be careful never to gorge myself in front of her.

Thus my binges usually took place on subway platforms or in parking lots or even while riding my bicycle. What I ate was usually something sweet: Baskin-Robbins ice cream (a pint at a time) or Pepperidge Farm Milano cookies (a bag at a time). I was always mortified that I might be spotted, sticky plastic spoon in hand, by someone I knew; a Phi Beta Kappa in her mid-twenties just didn't *do* things like gobble pints of ice cream out of a brown paper bag. However, I conveniently did my rationalizing *after* the fact. *While* I was sneak-eating, it seemed like a relatively harmless remedy for the career or romantic frustration I was experiencing. I wasn't falling-down drunk, I reasoned, and I wasn't shooting up heroin. But I *was* a compulsive overeater—and I was my mother's daughter far more than I cared to admit.

It took me years to comprehend, through self-help books, weight-loss classes, and finally psychotherapy, that it's impossible to grow up with a severely and chronically overweight parent without "inheriting" some of her low self-esteem—sort of like inferiority by association. While researching an article on this topic some years ago, I spoke with Philip Levendusky, Ph.D., a psychologist and the director of the eating-disorder program at Harvard's McLean Hospital in Belmont, Massachusetts. As he explained to me, "Having a fat parent may give you the feeling of being the product of someone less valued in society. Even if we're talking about your *mother*, there's still a stigma attached to *you*. If your feelings take the form of a fear of being overweight yourself—'Will this thing creep up and hit me, too? Will I turn out like *her*?'—then it's pretty straightforward. But it may be a lot more subtle—a sense that *nothing* you do is quite good enough."

I understood completely. My mother's failure to lose weight

despite countless attempts made *me* a failure of sorts, too—she was, after all, my earliest and most powerful role model. So even though I didn't have the severe weight problem she did, the 10-odd pounds I've repeatedly lost and gained since college have satisfied my innate desire to be like her—but not *too* much. Meanwhile, I've sought and found other ways to "fix" myself, becoming a perfectionist, a self-help junkie. Having a mother who followed a pattern of overeating/dieting/overeating/dieting led to *my* constant striving to "better" myself. My job, my income, my wardrobe, my apartment—nothing was ever good enough. I was always on the lookout for tips on improving my skin/my vocabulary/my job-hunting techniques/my investment returns—not to mention ways to drop those last 10 pounds.

"When the most important person in your world diets constantly, it's going to have an impact on you," Dr. Levendusky told me. "Watching her psychological torture—and, worse yet, her frustration when she fails to lose weight—may well lead you to believe you'll never achieve your own goals in life." Hence my never-ending quest for the perfect me.

And it's no accident that I keep as busy as I do. I travel a lot—whether that means an impromptu weekend jaunt to Philadelphia or two weeks in New Zealand—and I simply *do* more than most people I know. "Boy, you never slow down!" is a comment I hear constantly, and it's totally understandable: No one knows better than I my terror of becoming a prisoner of my own body.

My food-and-diet obsessions have even affected my career choices. Perhaps because I'd had so much experience nagging myself and my mother to lose weight, I accepted a job where I could put that skill to good use: as an editor at *Weight Watchers Magazine*. I remember that day in December 1980 when I was called for an interview by the then editor-in-chief. Judy was a sleek and beautiful woman, who, I was certain, never knew the anguish of passing up a cheese danish in favor of melba toast. At 132 pounds I was not fat, but next to her I *felt* it, and somehow I expected her to see me that way. Instead, Judy asked if I knew much about dieting or low-calorie menus. I smiled. Once I began rattling off some of the details of my Life with Mom, I knew I was a shoo-in.

A few weeks later the job was indeed mine, and I couldn't have been more pleased. But after a few years, I discovered that constantly hearing all that talk around the office of calories and carbohydrates and national obesity statistics was giving me a hard edge. Just as I had gotten disgusted over my mother's inability to buckle down and lose weight, I also began feeling that way about our readers. Because dieting and its attendant frustrations had been so much a part of my home life for three decades, my work environment had become too emotionally charged for me. Eventually I left—by then I was editor-in-chief—and went to work at another magazine. Today, years later, I can appreciate the irony that my mother's weight problem actually turned me into a diet "expert" and helped me land one of the best jobs I've ever had.

Mom may also have inadvertently been responsible for my winning the best mate I've ever had. Just as it's common for the child of an alcoholic to become emotionally involved with an alcoholic, I fell in love with Peter, a 5'8" writer who had formerly weighed 232 pounds—and as I later learned to my astonishment, secretly used to binge on ice cream in parking lots, just as I had done. By the time we met he was a svelte 162 and his eating problems were well in hand. But he *understood* me. It was a relief finally to be with someone who sympathized (and occasionally indulged me) when I peered longingly into the window of an all-you-can-eat restaurant. (My pencil-thin ex-boyfriend would have hurried me down the street with a fatherly, "Now, you don't need *that*!") Peter never lost his fondness for ice cream, but over the years he's done wonderfully in the weight-control department.

As for Mom, now a widow living on her own, she's still battling the bulge. When I go home to visit her these days, it's impossible to ignore all the food that's there—too much for a single-person household. Yet she continues her charade of Being on a Diet. Everything in her cupboards and refrigerator is marked "low-calorie" or "lite," and her night table is piled high with weight-loss books and videos. I see all this diet paraphernalia and can only wonder: What's the point? Thirty years ago, even 10, it would've made sense for her to try to drop some pounds. But despite a few potential benefits to her health (which has been all but wrecked because of her weight), I can't help wondering: Why bother *now*?

The answer, I suppose, is that she clings to the fantasy that somehow, someday she'll be a thin woman, for once in her life. She'll wear a form-fitting dress that doesn't require a breast-to-thigh corset beneath it, and she won't be out of breath after climbing a modest flight of stairs. My impulse is to laugh at the futility of it all—her desires have never been backed by commitment, so what can she expect? At the same time, I realize that she's far from unique; her dream is scarcely different from that of other overweight people who've simply managed to rein in their food demons better than she has.

Over the years my mother's weight has embarrassed me, worried me, frustrated me. Physically she's been an unfortunate role model, and she's unconsciously taught me to use food for all the wrong reasons. (There are *still* times when I can convince myself that a brownie will make everything okay.) But whatever else food may have represented to her, it always equaled love. Mom eats with abandon and cooks with abandon. She's brimming over with love, and she wants to share it with her adored family and friends. Regrettably, she hasn't been able to extend those expressions of love beyond the kitchen often enough. And, sadly, much of her self-love has dissolved into self-hate, symbolized by a body she's forever trying to escape.

It finally dawned on me that I was putting myself through a torment very similar to my mother's. After having done what amounted to a lifetime of research on the subject of dieting, I had an emotional and psychological breakthrough. It happened one day after I'd mentally beat myself up, as usual, for eating something I "shouldn't" have, in this case some cold noodles in sesame sauce. Why, I wondered, had I turned food into an excuse to punish myself constantly? Why couldn't I just eat it in reasonable amounts and *enjoy* it?

I knew the time had come for a drastic change in my thinking and my behavior. I started by making a list of the good and the bad in my life, in an effort to understand my compulsive overeating better. (Don't they always say making lists helps you figure things out?) My "good" list included my loving, stable relationship with Peter, who has always thought I was attractive and sexy regardless of my weight; a career I adore; good health; wonderful friends; and no real money worries. The list was, I noticed, fairly long. My "bad" list—headed by the familiar words "10 pounds overweight"—was quite short.

I realized I was being ridiculous to hate myself for not possessing a flat stomach or a tiny waist. I also decided that trying to get myself back to my college weight, given who I was *today*—a 40-year-old woman who loved to eat, disliked most forms of exercise, and had probably inherited some of her mother's extra fat cells—was unrealistic and cruel to my body and psyche. My whole pattern of inconsistent dieting, of focusing on every Frito and fish stick I put in my mouth—and agonizing over it later—had been making me neurotic. So I made the conscious decision to *stop dieting* and *relax* about my weight problem—which, after all, was never that much of a problem.

You can probably guess what happened next.

I started losing weight. Not *just* like that; it wasn't magic or anything. I merely found that as I became easier on myself and quit obsessing about the food I put in my mouth, I naturally put in less of it. As of this writing, I've got two or three pounds I'd like to lose. If I do, great. If I don't, I won't be the thinnest woman at the buffet table, but I may well be the most serene.

How I would love for Mom to know that serenity, too.

ABOUT THE AUTHOR

Linda Konner is an author, contributor to major magazines, university lecturer, and frequent talk-show guest.

She was associated with *Weight Watchers Magazine* for nearly five years, first as its managing editor and later as editor-in-chief, and she has written extensively on the subjects of food, diet, and health. Her byline has appeared in *The New York Times, Glamour, Redbook, Connoisseur, TV Guide, Seventeen, Woman's Day,* and many other publications, and she is the contributing entertainment editor of *Woman's World* magazine. Her books include *How to Be Successfully Published in Magazines* (St. Martin's Press) and three nonfiction works for young adults.

Konner has appeared on *Donahue, The Sally Jessy Raphael Show,* and countless radio programs, and she teaches magazine writing and marketing at colleges and writers' conferences around the country. She and her mate, Peter Filichia, live in New York City.